Essential Oils *for* Dental Health

A Holistic Guide to Oral Care and Treatment

Karin Opitz-Kreher
Jutta Schreiber, D.M.D.

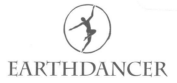

EARTHDANCER

AN INNER TRADITIONS IMPRINT

First edition 2022
Essential Oils for Dental Health
A Holistic Guide to Oral Care and Treatment
Karin Opitz-Kreher and Jutta Schreiber, D.M.D.

This English edition © 2022 Earthdancer GmbH
English translation © 2022 JMS books LLP
Editing by JMS books LLP (www.jmseditorial.com)

Originally published in German as:
Ätherische Öle für gesunde und schmerzfreie Zähne
World © 2018 Schirner Verlag, Darmstadt, Germany

Cover design: DesignIsIdentity.com
  Toothbrushes: Oleksandr Grechin, shutterstock.com;
  tea tree plant and flacon: Gummy Bear, shutterstock.com
Typesetting: DesignIsIdentity.com
Typeset in Minion

Printed and bound in China by Reliance Printing Co., Ltd.

ISBN 978-1-64411-578-7 (print)
ISBN 978-1-64411-579-4 (ebook)

Cataloging-in-Publication Data for this title is available from the Library of Congress.

Published by Earthdancer, an imprint of Inner Traditions
www.earthdancerbooks.com, www.innertraditions.com

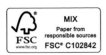

Contents

Introduction   7

The Relationship between Essential Oils and Teeth   11
  Fact Box: How we smell things   12
Why essential oils differ in quality   15
Methods of essential oil use   18
  Reflex zones on the hand   20
  Reflex zones on the feet   21
  Orange *(Citrus sinensis)*   23
  Lavender *(Lavandula angustifolia)*   25
  Applying essential oil to marma points   28
  Massaging trigger points   33
  Directing energy using mudras   37
  Dealing with fear   39

Maintaining Oral Health   43
The impact of healthy teeth on self-esteem *by Maria Kageaki*   46
Key essential oils and how to use them to support oral health   48
  Manuka *(Leptospermum scoparium)*   48
  Australian tea tree *(Melaleuca alternifolia)*   50
  Lemongrass *(Cymbopogon flexuosus)*   52
  Sage *(Salvia officinalis)*   53
  Oregano *(Oregano vulgare)*   54

Fact Box: Essential oils and homeopathic remedies 55

Clove *(Syzygium aromaticum)* 57

Treating oral health problems 58

Periodontal pockets and diabetes 58

Unhealthy teeth and rheumatism 60

Heart health 61

Hormones and dental issues 62

Periodontal problems 66

Oral candidiasis 71

Mouth sensitivity 75

Toothaches 77

Teething problems in infants 78

Fact Box: Using essential oils for babies and children 82

Wisdom teeth 83

Mouth ulcers 86

Cold sores 87

Dry mouth 90

Tooth decay 93

Fact Box: Coconut oil for a healthy, tooth-friendly diet 94

Oil pulling 95

Copaiba *(Copaifera reticulata)* 97

Bad breath 99

Myrtle *(Myrtus communis)* 102

Rosemary *(Rosmarinus officinalis)* 103

Spearmint *(Mentha spicata)* 104

Thyme *(Thymus vulgaris)* 105

Stress and teeth 106

Essential oil "stars"   108
  Rose *(Rosa damascena)*   109
  Lemon balm *(Melissa officinalis)*   112
  Sandalwood *(Santalum album)*   113

Epilogue   117

Recommended reading   119
Picture credits   120
About the authors   121

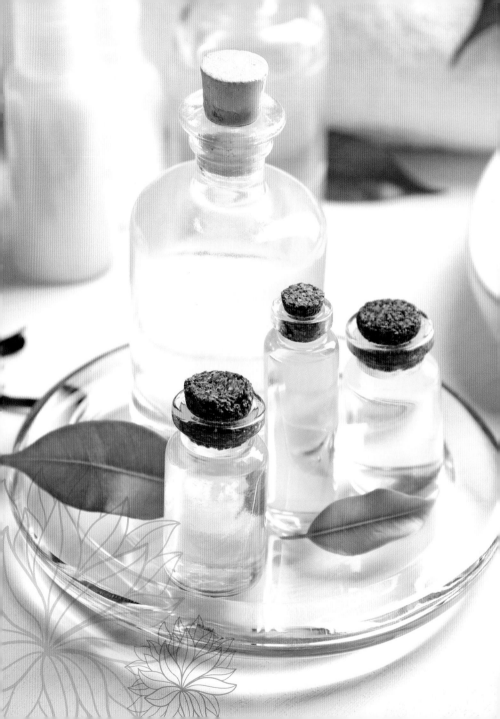

Introduction

I am surrounded by gold rings, beautiful bracelets, and shiny marbles in every color of the rainbow. Bouncing balls and yoyos fly in every direction, and small shiny cars race about.

My name is Jutta and these are my first memories of visiting a dentist.

Over the years I have realized that it was this toy box full of treasures, in which I was allowed to rummage after every visit, that drew me into this magical world, but it also had a strong and long-lasting influence on the way I thought about the dental clinic. I was always relaxed and looked forward excitedly to my dental appointment on each visit.

I also associate a very particular smell with these occasions, and it wasn't the typical odor of the nurse's office at school. Instead, I remember it as fruity and woody. Sadly, the dental surgery has long since closed, and I could never quite identify the precise source of the smell, but I remain convinced that emotions are closely connected with scents.

As a child born during the Second World War, my mother had always been unhappy about her teeth, which is why she always made sure that her children looked after theirs. Sitting in the waiting room almost began to feel like a weekly event. I had fillings, a few healthy teeth were pulled at an early age to make room for the others, and I lived with a range of different braces for many, many years.

I would sometimes hear my girlfriends complaining about being so scared of the dentist, but this was something new for me. While it was true that my whole mouth had always been extremely sensitive, and indeed still is, the routine nature of any dental appointments had always left a positive impression on me.

Indeed, so positive was the impression that I made dentistry my profession. I have been working in my own clinic for three decades now and have specialized in holistic dentistry for many years. I examine teeth and the masticatory system, not in isolation, but instead in the context of the whole body, mind, and spirit.

I have been excited about essential oils and their amazing applications for a number of years, and I couldn't imagine my clinic without them now. I hope you too will develop a new awareness and understanding of your mouth. Your lips, cheeks, tongue, palate, and teeth all deserve close attention. Wouldn't it be nice to feel relaxed and positive about your mouth? Concentrate on running your tongue around the whole of your inner cheeks, stroking the inside and outside of each individual tooth. Can you do it right away, without any difficulty? Over the years, the tongue sometimes becomes a little less agile, but with practice it can regain mobility. You will then notice changes in the mouth much more quickly and be able to take the appropriate action.

Suck in your cheeks and then blow them out again. Roll or purse your lips. Try pouting. This kind of short facial gymnastics session also helps to prevent the formation of wrinkles. Start your mouth awareness program today, and by getting to know your mouth in this playful and relaxed way, you will find that you are much calmer when you go to the dentist.

Unlike many of the current medicines in use in dentistry, essential oils are entirely natural. They are strong, potent substances and yet can be used without placing any unnecessary strain on the rest of the body.

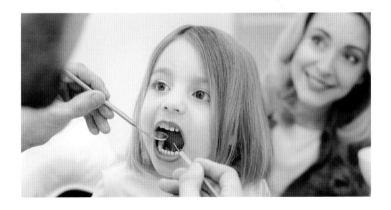

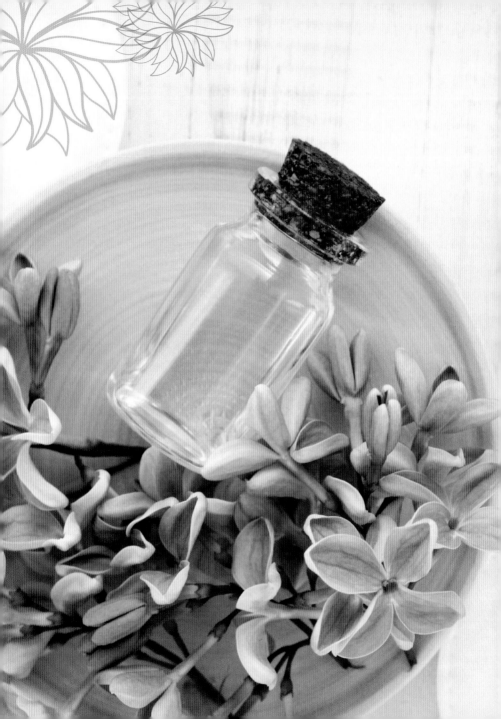

The Relationship between Essential Oils and Teeth

We have been taking advantage of the calming powers of essential oils in my clinic for twenty years now (writes Jutta), and for me it's the most natural thing in the world to have some relaxing citrus oil in the surgery. The first thing many patients notice when they walk into a dental clinic is its sterile smell, so it's no wonder that those who had bad childhood experiences at the dentist are immediately transported back in their memory and feel an associated chill down the spine.

If a patient is extremely tense, treatment under general anesthetic may be the only option, but I have firsthand experience of the difference essential oils can make in this regard. To be met by the welcoming, sunny fragrance of oranges as a patient opens the clinic door soon works its magic, putting a relaxed smile on their face before they even know it.

Initially, we mostly used essential oils for aromatherapy in the clinic, but over the last few years they have been increasingly used to help prepare and support a treatment. Essential oils can be applied externally but can also help with internal oral hygiene, and it's easy to make use of their positive properties in your own home.

It is my aim through the course of this book to introduce you to a number of essential oils that we use in our clinic both extensively and on a daily basis, and that can also be used at

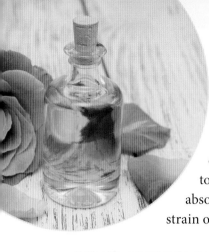

home to boost dental health or prepare for a visit to the dentist.

It is vital that the essential oils used are natural—synthetic scent molecules will certainly dock with the appropriate receptor cells, but they are not natural and when absorbed by the body, they put an enormous strain on the liver.

How we smell things

We are constantly being subjected to the odor of the things around us, often without realizing it, and yet the process of smelling something is actually fairly complex. Let's assume we can smell the intoxicating scent of a rose.

When we inhale, odor molecules reach the olfactory epithelium, a specialized tissue located on the roof of the nasal cavity, nearly 3 inches (7 cm) above and behind the nostrils. This tissue contains millions of olfactory receptor neurons, each one of which recognizes only very specific molecules.

When a receptor cell encounters a "matching" molecule, it triggers an electrical impulse that is transmitted (via the olfactory nerve) to the olfactory bulb, of which we have two, one above each nostril.

After further processing, the olfactory bulbs send the information to the brain, more specifically to the thalamus and limbic system (hippocampus and amygdala), where it plays a role in emotions, long-term memory, and learning.

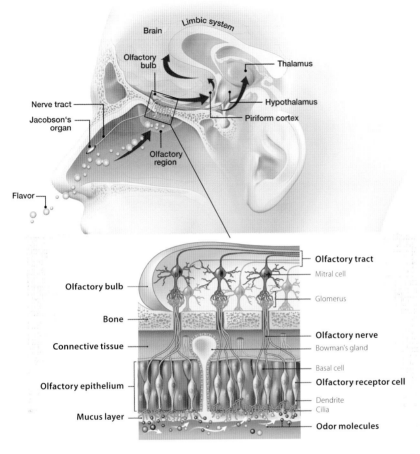

When we associate a pleasant memory with a particular scent, it helps to create emotional harmony. But when we smell burning, for example, our internal defenses kick into action and cause us to seek safety.

When our sense of smell is healthy, we are constantly perceiving odors and unconsciously evaluating whether we are safe or in danger.

If your dentist does not use essential oils to create a pleasant environment, take the matter into your own hands by putting a small drop of orange oil on your palms, rubbing them together, and then cupping both hands over your nose to breathe in the scent. If it is a high-quality essential oil, you will notice a change immediately. Everyone reacts slightly differently to particular scents, but most people associate the odor of oranges with freshness, sunshine, relaxation, and vacations.

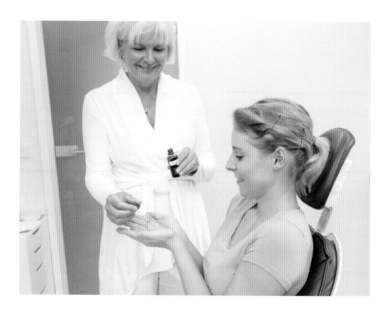

Why essential oils differ in quality

People often say that essential oils give them a headache, but why would that be the case?

Essential oils are not currently certified or approved by any regulatory body in the US, and it is as well to be aware that terms such as "therapeutic grade" or "pure" do not reflect the product's quality but are marketing terms to sell a product. An oil can be made from a 100 percent pure and natural product or an entirely synthetic one that has been artificially manufactured in a laboratory. A 100 percent pure oil may not necessarily be of the highest quality. Take cypress essential oil, for example, which contains 280 active ingredients that determine its effects and scent; the essential oil will contain all these components only if the cypress is distilled at the right temperature and pressure for exactly twenty-four hours. After twenty hours only twenty ingredients are extracted. However, increase this to twenty-six hours' distillation and the process destroys all the substances, rendering the oil wholly ineffective, and yet these are all up to 100 percent pure essential oils.

An essential oil is top quality only if it includes all the active ingredients from the plant and represents its essence. An orchestra is not all about a single violin; the key is the harmonious interplay between all the instruments.

Only a few manufacturers adhere to such high standards. Procedures such as spectroscopic analysis or gas chromatographic analysis are used to check whether the distillation process has worked. All kinds of unforeseen events can occur on the journey from planting and growing to harvesting and distilling the flowers.

I love going to Provence in the South of France for the lavender harvest (writes Karin). June 2017 was extremely hot and the lavender fields were unusually dry. The previous year only some plants had been so dry, while in other years the flowers were still closed or had opened by this time. But this year, as the plants had to make do with rainwater for irrigation, most of the flowers were dry. Our group went out to do some weeding. Weeds are no problem under normal conditions, as they have no scent and make up a small proportion of the harvest, but this year they were taking water away from the lavender.

The essential oils discussed in this book refer to high-quality products whose base plants were grown from seed, without the use of pesticides, herbicides, or fertilizers, and in soil that boasts good mineral levels. In an ideal world, the plants would come from sources located far from urban environments and would either be exposed to natural rainfall or irrigated with groundwater or purified water.

The way the plants are harvested is also key. Lavender is conventionally harvested using machines that shred the plants instantly. Any bee that happens to be on a flower has very little chance of survival, and a part of the essential oils is immediately lost due to its high volatility. Another mechanical harvesting option involves the lavender being "combed" and then snipped off. This is not as hard on the plant and bees can still fly away at any point.

Short distances from field to distillery are also important because mold can form during long journeys in transit, resulting in an oil of lower quality.

The art of distilling requires years of experience, considerable knowledge, and a certain knack. Even if the process between planting and harvest has gone well, distillation at too great a pressure or temperature can still reduce the quality.

Some people say that they cannot tolerate essential oils because the scent makes them feel sick. However, they are often surprised when they smell oils of the best quality and change their minds when they discover just how pleasant using them can actually be. I have seen the most convinced skeptic turn immediately into the most ardent fan.

Methods of essential oil use

There are a number of different approaches to the use of essential oils.

- The German school works principally with the sense of smell, such as with the oil being inhaled directly from the vial.
- The British school advocates mixing essential oils with a base oil and applying them to the body.
- The French school works with undiluted essential oils on the body, preferably applied to the reflex zones on the hands and feet.

Experiment to see which approach suits you best. As a general rule, the specific situation and the nature of the user will determine the preferred method.

If you're out and about, or even visiting the dentist, fill a roll-on bottle with a little carrier oil (a fatty oil such as almond, olive, or sesame oil) combined with a few drops of essential oil. Dab some on your wrists or neck while you're on the go.

For massage of the marma points (see p. 30) or the trigger points (see p. 33), it is advisable to mix essential oils with a carrier oil (for example, sesame, coconut, or olive oil).

Combining an essential oil with coconut or sesame oil allows it to be applied internally in the mouth; otherwise, undiluted essential oils can be too harsh on the gums. Do note that water intensifies the effects of the oils. Think of the burning sensation in the mouth after eating a hot chili pepper and how it makes the sensation worse when you drink water.

You can also use a drop of essential oil to massage the reflex zones on the soles of the feet or the palms of the hand. Since taking off shoes to massage your feet is generally not an option during the day, instead massage your hands, perhaps on a bus or train journey. When you massage your fingertips, for example, you focus on the reflex zones that correspond to your teeth. The people around you won't even notice.

When you are out and about, keep a small vial of essential oil to hand in your coat pocket or bag and inhale its scent briefly when you feel the need to relax—filling a room with the scent (such as in a public building) is not always appropriate.

Reflex zones on the hands

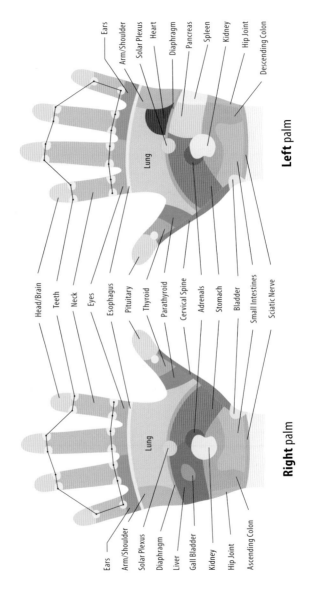

Left palm

Ears
Arm/Shoulder
Solar Plexus
Heart
Diaphragm
Pancreas
Spleen
Kidney
Hip Joint
Descending Colon

Head/Brain
Teeth
Neck
Eyes
Esophagus
Pituitary
Thyroid
Parathyroid
Cervical Spine
Adrenals
Stomach
Bladder
Small Intestines
Sciatic Nerve

Lung

Right palm

Ears
Arm/Shoulder
Solar Plexus
Diaphragm
Liver
Gall Bladder
Kidney
Hip Joint
Ascending Colon

Lung

Reflex zones on the feet

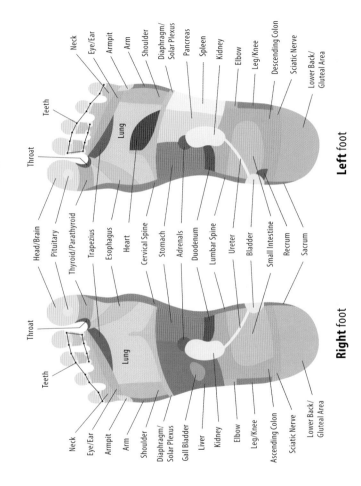

Right foot

Teeth
Throat
Neck
Eye/Ear
Armpit
Arm
Shoulder
Diaphragm/Solar Plexus
Gall Bladder
Liver
Kidney
Elbow
Leg/Knee
Ascending Colon
Sciatic Nerve
Lower Back/Gluteal Area

Lung

Head/Brain
Pituitary
Thyroid/Parathyroid
Trapezius
Esophagus
Heart
Cervical Spine
Stomach
Adrenals
Duodenum
Lumbar Spine
Ureter
Bladder
Small Intestine
Recrum
Sacrum

Left foot

Throat
Teeth
Neck
Eye/Ear
Armpit
Arm
Shoulder
Diaphragm/Solar Plexus
Pancreas
Spleen
Kidney
Elbow
Leg/Knee
Descending Colon
Sciatic Nerve
Lower Back/Gluteal Area

Lung

We routinely absorb a great number of substances that can be detrimental to us via our lungs and skin, as well as through our diet, water, and cosmetic products, so it makes sense to use products that are as natural and free of toxins as possible, particularly in oral and dental hygiene. Essential oils are effective and versatile in this respect, as they can be used in so many different ways to support a range of healthy functions throughout the body.

Essential oils have many effects and applications, bringing physical, emotional, and mental equilibrium. A plant that has a beneficial effect when applied orally can also sometimes influence other areas. As a rule, we always recommend using essential oils that have been distilled to retain all the active ingredients. Some plants are not yet available as an essential oil of this quality, in which case we recommend using the next best oil available; the point is to achieve the best results, rather than being dogmatic about which oil to use. The key is that everything is sourced naturally and is not synthetic.

Top tip for fear of the dentist:
Orange and lavender

Scientists at the University of Vienna discovered that the scent of oranges and lavender can help to deal with anxiety (although women were found to have responded to these scents far better than men). Studies at Mie University in Japan also confirmed this calming effect.

Orange *(Citrus sinensis)*
Botanical family:
Rutaceae (rue or citrus family)
Orange essential oil is cold pressed
from the peel.

Among its other properties, the scent of orange essential oil induces feelings of calm and cheer. It promotes a sense of well-being in most people, evoking sunny vacations in warm climates.

Do note that you should **not** apply orange oil to areas of skin that will be exposed to direct sunlight over the following twenty-four hours. It increases the skin's sensitivity to light and its susceptibility to sunburn. Routine application of the oil to the foot area works well.

Studies at the University of Arkansas have established that orange oil is effective against the *Staphylococcus aureus* bacterium, which should come as no surprise since plants form essential oils in order to protect themselves from viruses, bacteria, and mold. Distilled oils boast this protective property in even more concentrated form.

Other studies (such as those published in the *Journal of Advanced Biomedical Research*) report that the heart rate and cortisol levels of anxious patients were reduced when exposed to the scent of oranges, so reaching for a vial of orange essential oil in challenging, stressful situations should certainly help.

Top-quality orange oil still offers value for money and its versatility means it can be used in a variety of ways. Its scent can provide support in various everyday situations, and it helps with general stress reduction and in preparation for an appointment with the dentist. Some suggestions:

- Use with a diffuser as a room fragrance in the home.
- A roll-on (0.17 fl oz/5 ml) neutral carrier oil such as almond or jojoba oil, plus 5 drops of orange oil) for dabbing on the wrist.
- Rub a drop onto your palms and cup your hands over your nose to inhale the scent. Note how your breathing and posture slowly relax.
- Massage of the marma points (see p. 30) or trigger points (see p. 33).

Lavender *(Lavandula angustifolia)*
Botanical family:
Lamiaceae (labiates)

Lavender essential oil is obtained through steam distillation of the flower tips of the plant.

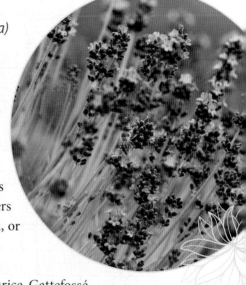

A perfectly balanced lavender oil is obtained from a combination of flowers that have withered, are still in bloom, or are small, unopen buds.

We have French chemist René-Maurice Gattefossé (1881–1950) to thank for contemporary interest in the benefits of essential oils. After growing up in a family of perfumers, he discovered their healing power after he was badly injured in a laboratory explosion and decided to try lavender oil on the wound, enabling him to experience its regenerative properties at first hand.

Lavender oil is extremely effective for skin problems. It can be applied topically to cold sores or herpes to support the healing process (it doesn't burn).

Lavender oil boosts beta waves in the brain (as demonstrated by studies at the University of Miami), thereby delivering deeper relaxation.

When buying lavender oil, be sure to look for the botanical name *Lavandula angustifolia* on the label (common name, true or English lavender). The flowers of each plant in a field of true lavender look a little different—some may be deep violet and others more of a light pastel shade. Fields of true lavender tend not to be very spectacular, unlike the dramatically deep purple meadows of "bouquet lavender," the type you would buy from a florist. The latter is grown to be tied into bunches and each plant is identical to the next, the appearance being more important than any active ingredients.

Lavender oil can be found for sale in markets at apparently tempting prices, but be aware that it could be a blend or even not lavender at all. It may be lavandin, a related plant, whose scent is more familiar since it is cheaper and therefore often used in washing powders and soaps. Lavandin is valued for its cleansing properties but lacks the calming effects of lavender.

Many farmers prefer to grow lavandin rather than lavender for economic reasons. It is a hybrid (unable to reproduce) and is grown from cuttings, so all the plants look identical. There can be up to three panicles on each stem, meaning that the yield for lavandin can be as much as 8–10 gallons per acre (90–120 liters per hectare), while lavender with just one panicle (which is also smaller in size) would produce only one or two gallons per acre (20 liters per hectare). Lavandin is also not susceptible to *Cixiidae* planthoppers that transmit a fungus that then shrinks the lavender. Things reached a crisis point in the region of Provence in France a few years ago when many lavender fields had to be burned to prevent an epidemic. To avoid using artificial pesticides, the farmers employ a mixture of clay and water that combats pests naturally, although the best prevention is to practice crop rotation. Alternately planting lavender and einkorn wheat, an ancient grain variety, is better for the soil, and good soil produces healthy, robust plants.

A combination of orange and lavender oils enhances mood and induces relaxation, both of which can be a great help when visiting the dentist. It is also an effective combination for use in the dental clinic since most patients enjoy both fragrances.

Applying essential oil to marma points

Marma therapy, a treatment involving the marma points (specific energy points on the body), is a pleasant way to induce a feeling of relaxation and reduce anxiety. It can be used both in the office and at home. Oils extracted from geranium, mandarin, lavender, cedarwood, or sandalwood are old favorites for this. In my clinic (writes Jutta), we use the following homemade oil mixtures.

Stabilization and acceptance

5 drops of lavender essential oil
15 drops of mandarin essential oil
10 drops of sandalwood essential oil
5 drops of cedarwood essential oil
in 1 fl oz (30 ml) jojoba oil

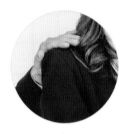

Relaxation

5 drops of wintergreen essential oil
4 drops of juniper essential oil
5 drops of lemon essential oil
2 drops of chamomile essential oil
8 drops of mandarin essential oil
in 1 fl oz (30 ml) sesame oil

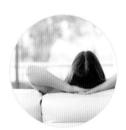

8 drops of rosewood essential oil
2 drops of lavender essential oil
2 drops of geranium essential oil
2 drops of sandalwood essential oil
1 drop of blue chamomile essential oil
1 drop of cardamom essential oil
in 1 fl oz (30 ml) jojoba oil

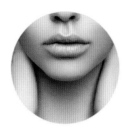

Marma therapy is practiced as an independent form of therapy within Ayurveda. It identifies a total of 107 massage points. I put two or three drops of the oil mixture onto my palms and those of my patient. We both rub our hands together briefly, then cup them over our noses to breathe in and enjoy the fragrance.

Now take a seat, make yourself comfortable, sit up straight, and practice some box breathing (also known as square breathing). Breathe in as you count to four in your head. Hold your breath for a count of four and breathe out, counting to four again. Hold your breath for another count of four and begin the sequence again. Repeat five or six times. It will help you to get in the mood, prepare, and relax.

You are now ready to massage your own marma points. I can tell you from experience that gently holding or pressing the marma points is enough to get the energy flowing.

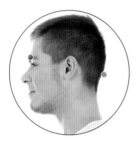

Gently press the "power band" on the nape of your neck with one hand and your third eye with the middle finger of the other. The power band is the region where the head reaches the first cervical vertebra. The third eye is on the forehead between the eyebrows, level with the pineal gland.

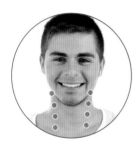

Now gently press the neck marmas. These are four areas on each side of the neck along the carotid artery. This will also help support the thyroid gland. These points are effective when you are distressed or have an emotional blockage, something "stuck in the throat," metaphorically speaking. The stomach, small intestine, and colon are all brought into harmony, the nape of the neck relaxes, and the throat will clear of mucus.

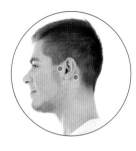

Now gently press the ear marmas. These include a point in front of the tragus and one behind the ear. Pressing both of these at once is good for neck problems or anxiety. These points work in a similar way to the stabilization and acceptance oil (see p. 28). Whenever you feel hesitant or unsure about something, pressing these two points should help you to feel more grounded and on an even keel.

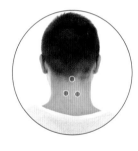

Along with those practicing many other professions, dentists frequently suffer from severe muscle tension across the neck and shoulder area. This tension can be treated with splint therapy, complemented by gently pressing the neck marmas. These are three points that are the seat of our anxiety: two at the junction of the head and the cervical spine to the right and left of the vertebrae and one in a central furrow beneath the back of the head. Pressing these points will boost self-confidence and self-awareness, helping you to relax and clear your head.

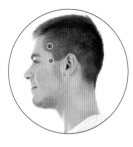

Finally, the temple marmas can be used to reduce the grinding and clenching of teeth, and to help counteract overexertion and feelings of anger and rage. Relax all the facial muscles by pressing the points located midway between the corner of the eye and the point where the top of the ear meets the head and three finger widths above this.

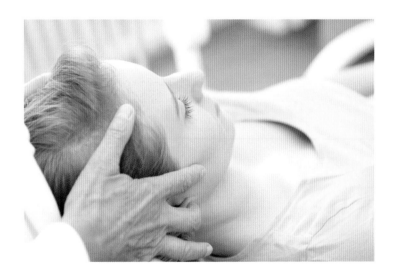

Massaging trigger points

Many people process stress by clenching, grinding, or chattering their teeth at night. This can put excessive strain on the muscles and joints within the masticatory system (and elsewhere). This tension can even be transmitted via the neck and shoulders to the upper and lower back area, hips, knees, or feet, resulting in problems that are far removed physically from their causal point.

Trigger points reveal chronic overloading of the muscular system (producing hyper-tensed muscles or knots in the muscles). The German Pschyrembel clinical dictionary defines these as stimulation points that cause pain (including referred pain) when touched. These sensitive areas have great diagnostic value for therapists.

One such impairment of the joints of the jaw is also known as craniomandibular dysfunction (CMD). Those affected generally report non-specific pain in the jaw area that can also impair speech, drinking, or chewing. Problems with the jaw should always be addressed by a dentist to prevent risks to health.

In the dental clinic, the cause of the pain (incorrect bite alignment, ocular malposition, abnormal foot position, and so on) will be established with a range of tests. If the cause is located within the masticatory system, it can be mitigated with splint therapy, which your dentist would handle.

In order to relieve the strain on the trigger points around the jaw, I apply complementary matrix rhythm therapy (writes Jutta). A device with a vibrating head is used to stimulate and harmonize the vibrations of the tissue and cells from 8 to 12 Hertz (Hz).

The strain on trigger points can be relieved and muscular tension soothed through self-massage of the *Musculus masseter* (masseter muscle) area, one of the four muscles used for chewing. This muscle arises from the zygomatic bone and is inserted into the angle of the mandible and the mandibular ramus (corner of the jaw). In addition to actually clenching the teeth, it also permits the lower jaw to move laterally and longitudinally to chew food into smaller pieces. This muscle reacts particularly sensitively to emotional and mental strain. Stress, inner tension, false ambition, and a sense of hopelessness can result in unconscious overload.

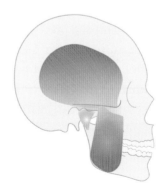

- Trigger points in the upper half of the muscle can induce pain in the upper jaw that can resemble sinusitis. They can also cause the pain of toothache in the upper molars.
- Trigger points in the central/lower area can cause pain in the lower jaw and toothache in the lower molars.
- Trigger points in the lower section often lead to head pain similar to a tension headache.
- Trigger points in deeper structures can cause pain in the mandibular joint and ears, even leading to tinnitus.

The best way to find your masseter muscle is to place it under pressure by clenching your teeth firmly. If you now trace the structures of the muscle with your fingertips, you will find areas that are painful, hard, and difficult to move. Massage these points with the jaw muscle relaxation oil mixture given on the following page.

Press gently on the painful area with two or three fingers, rotating gently clockwise as you move your jaw. Make chewing movements, side-to-side movements, or rotate your lower jaw. You should feel some relief after repeating this a few times.

Loosening up

7 drops of pine essential oil
3 drops of wintergreen essential oil
3 drops of immortelle essential oil
2 drops of peppermint essential oil
2 drops of clove essential oil
in 1 fl oz (30 ml) sesame oil

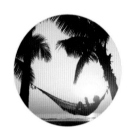

Directing energy using mudras

Mudras, gestures made using the hands or fingers that can guide the flow of energy in the body, have also proved useful in dental treatment. In the West we know them mostly as a part of yogic practice, but this positional use of the hands (and feet) is widespread in India in particular.

Many patients are unsure what to do with their hands as they sit in the dentist's chair and mudras provide a welcome solution. The following are some of the mudras that promote relaxation and dispel anxiety, but there are, of course, many more.

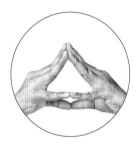

Hakini mudra

For the Hakini mudra, gently place the fingertips of your hands together (thumb to thumb, index finger to index finger, and so on). This should deepen your breathing and loosen up the entire body. Oxygen is fed to the brain as you begin to relax.

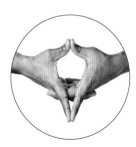

Uttarabodhi mudra

Gently interlock your fingers, extending your index fingers and thumbs so that the tips touch, with your thumbs pointing back toward your body. This mudra brings relaxation and brightens the mood, and can also be used to fight anxiety and panic.

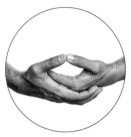

Dhyana mudra

The Dhyana mudra is the classic finger pose adopted during meditation. Both hands are laid in the lap like a bowl, with the left placed over the right. The tips of both thumbs touch to form the shape of a handle. This will help you to find inner peace.

Durga mudra

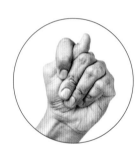

For the Durga mudra, close your hands into fists and tuck each thumb between its respective index and middle finger. This mudra helps you to deal with feelings of anxiety and panic. It is wise not to fight such feelings but to accept them as part of us, as a signal. Using the help of the mudra to get through a situation generating such feelings signifies that a step in the right direction has already been taken. The mudra provides the support required to bolster courage and calm your mind. Breathe out for longer as you hold the mudra.

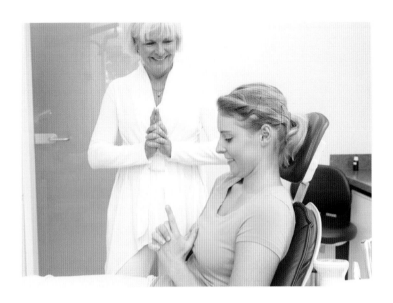

Dealing with fear

I learned an exciting technique to deal with fear of the dentist from emotions coach Caroline Adelskamp (writes Karin). It is known as the Wingwave® method and can be used to "wave away" stress, fear, and emotional blockages.

According to the WHO (World Health Organization), half of us suffer from stress, and for one in ten this involves crippling side effects that include blackouts, palpitations, tremors, sweating fits, and nausea.

Most of what we experience during the day is then worked through during our nightly dream phase. The unconscious eye movements during sleep (the REM phase) induce different areas of the brain to work together, separating the emotions attached to an experience from the detail of what happened. We may remember that a heated argument with a neighbor took place, for example, but no longer feel any of the associated anger, which has now dissipated like smoke. The emotion has been processed.

However, this processing does not always work out and issues can become rooted in the emotional brain, forming connections that have nothing to do with the original experience. Seemingly harmless situations can give rise to fear of flying, for example, or claustrophobia, exam fever, anxiety in the dentist's surgery or in traffic, and other emotional blockages.

Wingwave® is based on the latest brain research and in principle uses the same technique as the brain to relieve stubborn feelings of stress while a patient is awake. The root cause of the emotional blockage is ascertained with a muscle test, and patients then concentrate on the emotion that is troubling them while following the coach's rapid hand movements (like a wave) with their eyes. This identifies the stressors and decouples them from the emotions.

Just three sessions have proved to be sufficient for dealing with a previously blocked situation (for example, an appointment with the dentist).

We have now introduced a number of ways in which patients can be helped to relax in the dental surgery, although the best solution is, of course, to follow a regime of preventive care and good oral hygiene. That way your only visit will be to attend for a checkup!

One request: parents of a newborn baby should not put a pacifier or spoon in their own mouth before giving it to their baby. There is a risk of passing on their own oral microbiome, which is not conducive to their child's oral hygiene.

Healthy teeth and firm gums are also rooted in a healthy gut and a robust immune system. You can achieve this with regular exercise, a healthy diet, a low-stress lifestyle, and sufficient contact with the natural world, but try to pay attention to your emotional balance too, as repressed emotions can cause excessive acidification of the tissues. Applying pressure to marma points and using breathing techniques may help.

If you find you enjoy daily treatment with essential oils produced from plants, you will soon notice the physical, emotional, and mental equilibrium that these can bring. Their versatility means they can be used in so many different ways.

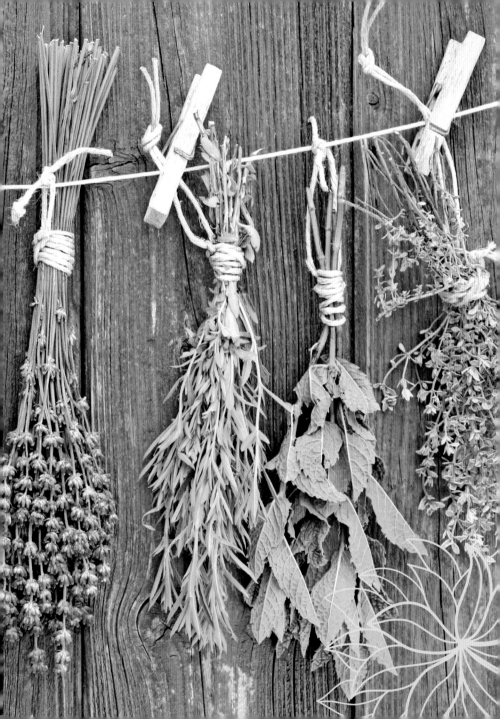

Maintaining Oral Health

With good preventive care, a six-monthly checkup at the dentist should only entail a short visit, possibly detecting just the smallest of cavities before they have the chance to become more problematic. Professional cleaning maintains oral health, and a dental hygienist can advise on the correct toothbrush, the most effective brushing technique, and the use of any other equipment such as interdental brushes and dental floss.

The tongue itself reveals a great deal about a person's state of health, pinpointing regions that could be under strain (gut, liver, or gall bladder) but is often neglected. It is therefore worth taking the time to check the tongue on a daily basis. Cleaning the tongue with a special brush and essential oils helps to maintain its health (see also p. 99).

Oil pulling derives from Ayurvedic healing and involves rinsing the mouth first thing in the morning with a teaspoon of sesame oil for at least five minutes, after which the oil is spat out into a paper towel and thrown into the trash (rather than simply spat into a sink, as the oil may thicken and ultimately clog pipes) and the mouth thoroughly rinsed with water. This draws out toxins and firms up the gums, and we recommend that patients add a few drops of grapefruit essential oil to the sesame oil to enhance its effects.

Products that contain essential oils obtained from cloves, rosemary, eucalyptus, spearmint, vetiver, or lemon are recommended for oral care at home. These support the alkaline environment in the mouth and leave it feeling clean and hygienic. Test strips available from pharmacies can be used to check the pH levels of your saliva and urine from time to time. When analyzing such test results, it is helpful to be aware that more acids are excreted from the body at certain times than at others, and that the alkaline level of your urine is likely to be higher at certain times of the day. Urine tends to be more alkaline around 4am, 10am, 4pm, and 10pm. More acids are excreted around 1am, 7am, 1pm, and 7pm.

Acids can still predominate in the mouth even if the urine is alkaline, however, and essential oils help greatly in promoting a healthy oral environment.

We also mix our own polishing pastes in the clinic in order to avoid chemical additives, using a mixture of zeolite (a powder of volcanic origin), clary sage oil, and calendula toothpaste.

The interdental spaces are cleaned with a small brush dipped in our oil mixtures, which we emulsify in order to reach the base of the gingival pockets (the base of the gums).

If inflammation of the gums does occur, it is very important to treat it. What may be regarded as just some slight bleeding of the gums should be taken seriously. Many older people suffer from periodontitis (a disease of the periodontium, which holds the teeth in place), but most underestimate just how dangerous this condition can be for other organs in the body. By the same token, diseases affecting the whole body can also influence mouth health.

Numerous studies have shown a connection between periodontitis and other serious conditions, including cardiac and circulatory disease, arteriosclerosis, diabetes, stroke, gastritis, and even premature birth or birth complications.

Inflammation is easy to miss and often causes no pain, making it doubly hard to visualize the extent. If it were possible to add together all the inflamed areas of a person suffering from generalized periodontitis, the infected area could well be about the size of their palm. If they had an infection of a similar size on their leg, for example, they would certainly not ignore it.

The impact of healthy teeth on self-esteem
by Maria Kageaki

Healthy teeth represent vigor and suggest a vitality that helps one to negotiate life successfully. To "get one's teeth into things" means having the strength and power to get on in life, an important feature of the journey to healthy teeth. Solid self-esteem has a direct effect on dental health.

A person's daily diet has significant consequences for the health of their teeth, which are greatly affected by the acid-base homeostasis in the mouth (the balance between the acids and bases/pH). Stress can also result in over-acidification and an increase in the urge to eat sweet things, making it a major cause of dental caries (decay). The first occurrence of caries in a child marks the preliminary stage in a general demineralization of the body. It is an indication that certain changes in diet and lifestyle are required.

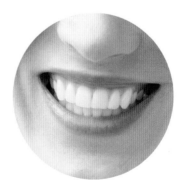

Teeth demineralize but live teeth can also be remineralized; thorough chewing effectively supports the calcification of teeth and jawbone when the appropriate minerals are available. Alongside a diet rich in vegetables, a number of other factors support remineralization, including sunlight (Vitamin D3), physical activity, and a stable acid/alkaline balance. It is therefore very important to protect the teeth. The cost of a healthy diet is minimal in comparison to the incalculable value of general physical well-being.

Key essential oils
and how to use them to support oral health

Why does a plant produce essential oils? It uses them for protection from potential harm within its environment, from foreign invaders such as fungus, bacteria, viruses, and parasites. These essential oils possess the very properties required to ensure our own dental hygiene.

For example, to curb unwanted oral flora, essential oils can be mixed into coconut or sesame oil (so-called carrier oils). This dilutes the essential oils, which can otherwise be too strong, and makes them easier to apply.

Manuka *(Leptospermum scoparium)*
Botanical family: *Myrtaceae* (myrtles)
The leaves and stems are steam-distilled to make manuka essential oil.

Manuka will probably be familiar through its connection with the manuka honey produced in New Zealand and Australia. Manuka is prized for the excellent quality of the substances it contains. The Maori, the indigenous people of New Zealand, call the shrub "mānuka." It is, in fact, a shrub-type tree that resembles the Australian tea tree. Like cajeput, niaouli, and kanuka, it is often traded as "tea tree," although the fragrance of manuka oil is a little warmer and milder than that of Australian tea tree oil.

Manuka has powerful cleansing properties and studies have shown it to be highly effective against antibiotic-resistant organisms. Its powerful effect against inflammatory processes, fungal infection, and bacterial problems should be emphasized in this respect. Some bacteria form a protective slimy layer known as a biofilm to shield against attack. Scientific studies have shown that manuka can destroy this biofilm. This is a key property, as this layer of mucus must be breached in order to fight the bacteria.

Manuka has also been shown to help people who suffer from stress or anxiety.

Australian tea tree
(Melaleuca alternifolia)
Botanical family:
Myrtaceae (myrtles)
The leaves are steam-distilled to
make tea tree essential oil.

This evergreen tree with white bark grows largely in Australia. Its young branches look as though they are covered in fine hair. The Australian tea tree flourishes along the rivers and marshes of the states of New South Wales and Queensland, where it grows to a height of up to 23 feet (7 meters).

The essential oil obtained from the tea tree is the plant's most widely known application, but Aboriginal Australians, Australia's First Peoples, would use the leaves to bind wounds or to drink as an infusion. Tea tree oil possesses powerful cleansing properties due to its very high levels of terpenes (which also give it its powerful scent), and this is what makes it effective for oral use. Add a drop to water for gargling or rinsing the mouth.

The cleansing properties of tea tree oil are highly valued for treating teeth or gum problems, and it can help with sinus and lung issues while also being kind to the skin. The oil can even treat fungal infections.

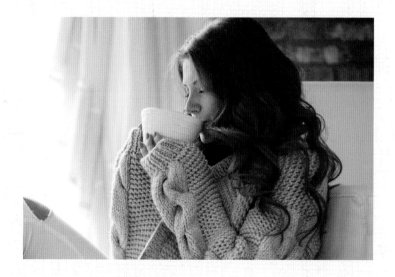

Lemongrass *(Cymbopogon flexuosus)*
Botanical family:
Poaceae (grasses/sweet grasses)
Lemongrass essential oil is obtained
through steam distillation of the grass.

This robust evergreen grass originated in India and can grow to a height of up to 6 feet (2 meters). Lemongrass is a familiar herb in Asian cooking and is also drunk as a tea. It has a fresh, lemony scent that adds a finishing touch to the flavor of many dishes. The fragrance of the essential oil is fresh and tangy and in medical studies it has demonstrated strong cleansing properties. When laboratory tests studied the performance of ninety-one essential oils against *Staphylococcus aureus* (a cause of skin and other infections) in 2008, lemongrass was found to be the only oil that would completely halt the growth of the test culture.

Studies have also shown lemongrass to be of use against fungal infections.

In addition to its cleansing powers, it has calming properties, and its scent promotes mental acuity and clarity.

Lemongrass also stimulates the circulation and the lymphatic system.

Chao, P. et al.: Inhibition of methicillin-resistant *Staphylococcus aureus* by essential oils. In: *Flavour and Fragrance Journal*. Wiley 2008, p. 444–449.

Sage *(Salvia officinalis)*

Botanical family: *Lamiaceae* (labiates)
Sage essential oil is obtained through
steam distillation of the leaves.

The sage plant is native to the Mediterranean and is especially prevalent in Croatia, Spain, and France, although subspecies occur worldwide. The leaves are used as a herb in rich dishes or to make tea.

In the ancient world, sage was considered a holy plant by both the Greeks and the Romans, and it was also used in medieval Europe to treat issues in the mouth and throat.

Sage essential oil has powerful cleansing properties and makes a good mouth rinse. Its fragrance has a strengthening and revitalizing effect and helps to calm anxiety.

Do note that this oil should **not** be used by women during pregnancy or when breast-feeding, as it inhibits milk flow and can even cause ablactation (cessation of milk secretion). Sage can also affect the hormonal system and may influence estrogen, progesterone, and testosterone levels. Sage oil should not be used in the event of epilepsy or high blood pressure.

Oregano *(Oregano vulgare)*

Botanical family:
Lamiaceae (labiates)

Oregano essential oil is obtained through steam distillation of the leaves.

Oregano, also known as wild marjoram, is a tough herb that grows wild throughout Europe.

Fresh or dried oregano leaves are mostly used as a culinary herb or in healing, but the essential oil is also highly regarded. Oregano has been prized as a medicinal herb since the Middle Ages and is even cited in the works of Hildegard of Bingen, a visionary medieval healer.

Oregano is beneficial for the respiratory and digestive systems, promoting healthy gut flora, and is capable of destroying bacterial biofilm. Its cleansing properties are due to its carvacrol and thymol content.

Because of its high phenol levels, oregano oil is classed as one of the "hot" essential oils. This means that it can be an irritant when used undiluted, so mixing it with a fatty carrier oil is advisable, especially for internal applications.

Essential oils and homeopathic remedies

Expert opinion is divided on the use of essential oils in homeo-pathy. Some specialists maintain that oils such as peppermint may superimpose themselves on and/or expunge the informa-tion carried by a homeopathic substance. Other strong herbs such as oregano and thyme should therefore also be avoided when taking homeopathic remedies.

In each case, it is advisable to discuss the situation in depth with your physician or naturopath.

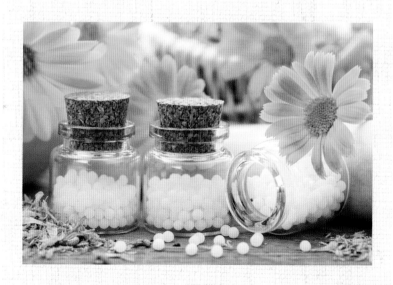

The essential oils mentioned so far generally have an intense fragrance, but people who find their strong and distinctive flavors unpleasant for internal use may prefer to opt for orange oil instead (see p. 23). Alongside its very fresh taste, orange oil also boasts a strong cleansing effect.

Anyone with concerns about whether orange oil is suitable for dental use should rest assured that it has nothing to do with orange juice, which certainly does attack teeth enamel. The essence is extracted from the peel and has no negative effects.

Before brushing my teeth (writes Karin), I like to add a drop of orange essential oil to a natural toothpaste that contains no synthetic substances. This makes the mouth feel even fresher. Do not use conventional toothpaste in this instance, as its chemical ingredients may clash with the essential oil, causing the body to embark immediately on its detoxification processes.

Clove *(Syzygium aromaticum)*
Botanical family:
Myrtaceae (myrtles)
Essential oil is extracted from the
flower buds and stems of the
clove plant.

This evergreen tree can reach heights
of up to 33 feet (10 meters) and forms
small flower buds that turn into cloves.
The best quality plants came originally
from the Indonesian Maluku Islands, where
the indigenous people were renowned for their
good health. However, when Dutch seafarers arrived
and destroyed the trees in the 16th century, the islanders' resistance to disease waned and many fell victim to illnesses that had been introduced by the Europeans.

Cloves were used widely in the Middle Ages and were prized by natural healer Hildegard of Bingen, as well as by physicians in China and India. Cloves were used in dental medicine in particular and today dried cloves are a familiar home remedy for toothache. The active ingredient is eugenol, which has a mild local anesthetic effect.

Clove essential oil is classed as a "hot" oil and should always be diluted for use.

Do note that clove oil has anticoagulant properties.

Treating oral health problems

Periodontal pockets and diabetes

Our knowledge of the connection between teeth and health goes back millennia. An Ancient Babylonian clay tablet from 800 BCE records this finding in cuneiform script: "If his teeth have darkened, his disease will be long-lasting."

The reciprocal relationship between systemic disease (such as diabetes mellitus) and periodontal disease has now been confirmed. Diabetics are up to three times more likely than healthy people to develop periodontitis and, by the same token, those with advanced periodontitis are at significantly higher risk of contracting diabetes. The exact mechanism of this relationship is yet to be conclusively explained.

If type 2 diabetics have well-balanced blood sugar levels, however, their risk of periodontitis is not increased. Diabetes patients certainly do seem to derive great benefit from periodontal therapy and the regular cleaning of risk areas for oral inflammation.

Cinnamon essential oil can address several issues at once. It has powerful cleansing properties and supports the healthy function of the pancreas. A mouthwash comprising a drop of cinnamon oil diluted in sesame oil (as a carrier oil) can be used to counteract periodontitis and help stave off diabetes (but remember not to swallow any!).

Ready-made mouthwashes containing essential oils are also available, derived from cinnamon, clove, rosemary, eucalyptus, lemon, spearmint, peppermint, and vetiver. These can be powerful, especially when you consider that each individual essential oil can contain between 300 and 500 different substances. The chances are high that these will include a natural active ingredient that can combat the bacteria responsible.

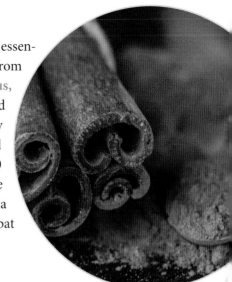

Unhealthy teeth and rheumatism

The 18th-century American physician Benjamin Rush reported how one patient's arthritis improved after extraction of their infected teeth, but studies demonstrating a connection between inflammatory rheumatic disorders and periodontitis have been published only in recent years. People with serious periodontitis are 2.5 times more likely to develop rheumatism than those without it.

In the same way, it has been demonstrated that patients with rheumatoid arthritis are at greater risk of developing periodontitis, hence the recommendation that rheumatism sufferers have their teeth professionally cleaned and treated every three months. In our experience, this may indeed have a positive effect on the severity, and development of, rheumatoid arthritis.

It is a good idea to complement the treatment of inflammatory processes with an oil such as frankincense or copaiba. These oils are applied to the skin and are at their most effective when absorbed through the soles of the feet or the palms of the hand.

In addition, both essential oils have a rejuvenating effect on the skin. Combined with coconut or sesame oil, they make a good facial treatment. The essential oils enter the bloodstream through the skin and are transported to wherever they can provide support.

Heart health

The many root causes of coronary heart problems include an unhealthy lifestyle, genetic predisposition, high blood pressure, excessive stress, and depression. Unhealthy teeth clearly also have an effect on the heart, and studies of heart attack patients have identified periodontitis cells from the mouth deposited as plaque in the heart (cardiac) veins, which then become congested or blocked with plaque over time.

Studies have also shown that successful periodontitis therapy improves heart vessel function and typically reduces inflammation levels in the blood. Dental care can, therefore, have a distinctly positive effect on cardiac health.

Here too, suitable essential oils can successfully complement other treatments, for example, tea tree oil for oral hygiene. For a more targeted use of oils, an individual's bacterial makeup can be tested. Bacterial biomes can differ greatly from person to person.

Hormones and dental issues

Life does not always go as smoothly as we would like. For example, at certain times our bodies face periods of physical upheaval, such as during puberty, pregnancy, and the menopause. Control hormones often "go crazy" during these times, and it is not just the cells of the body as a whole that need to reregulate themselves. The effects are often noticed first in the gums, which become swollen, inflamed, and turn red, bleeding at the slightest touch. In our experience, intensive treatment with oils extracted from sage, clove, thyme, oregano, tea tree, or lemongrass can offer an effective complementary therapy.

The hormonal system is fairly complex (writes Jutta). I always try to explain it in terms of an organogram, a graphic representation of a company's structure. Let's call the body "Me Inc." The hypothalamus is the CEO, under whose leadership is the Executive Board of the pituitary gland and the pineal gland located in the brain. When these glands are working properly, everything also works smoothly in the departments below them (thyroid gland, thymus gland, pancreas, adrenal glands, gonads, and so on). And the gonads (ovaries and testicles) indicate how the brain is functioning—the more vigorous the gonads, the more active the brain and the cerebral glands.

In addition to the way our bodies develop and age, a number of different external influences can also play a part in disrupting our hormonal system:

- Microplastics affect the gonads and/or the sex hormones.
- Eating meat from animals raised by factory farming methods affects the growth hormones (due to the substances used in this type of farming), which can result in greater susceptibility to cancer. This includes the stress hormones generated in the animal when it is slaughtered.
- The high proportion of blue light emitted by artificial lighting and screens affects the pineal gland and melatonin production, which can disrupt sleep patterns.
- Fluoride, electrosmog, and heavy metals affect the brain and the cerebral glands on a general basis.
- Long-term stress at work and in daily life depletes the adrenal glands over time.
- A diet that includes too many sweet things and so-called empty carbohydrates can upset the pancreas.
- The burden of emotional stress on the liver can also have repercussions for the thyroid gland, since hormones produced by the thyroid gland are metabolized and transformed in the liver.

For a more precise picture of your own current hormone levels (in order to manage them in a more targeted manner), ask your physician or alternative practitioner to carry out a saliva test.

Certain essential oils are worth mentioning in particular for the great support they provide to the body's hormonal system. They can boost blood circulation in the brain, allowing an increase in the production of neurotransmitters and hormones, helping to improve general well-being.

- For the cerebral glands: frankincense, sandalwood, and cedarwood essential oils
- For the thyroid gland: myrrh and myrtle essential oils
- For the pancreas: cinnamon and ocotea essential oils
- For the adrenal glands: nutmeg and black pepper essential oils
- For the gonads: clary sage, geranium, and yarrow essential oils

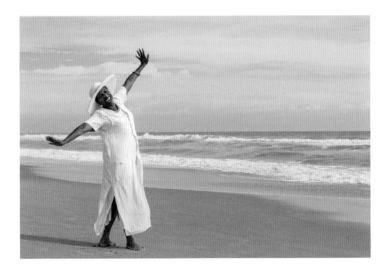

Plants produce essential oils for self-protection and to attract insects with the scent. In this respect, for the plant the oils are rather like our own hormonal and immune systems. As part of nature ourselves, our bodies are able to interact well with these natural oils.

Versatile essential oils can help in a wide range of areas. However, since we are all different, their effects vary slightly from person to person, with the oils' ingredients interacting with each of us in different ways.

When the body's hormones are disrupted or out of balance, it is important to follow an alkaline diet, to take care of the digestive system, to detoxify and/or purge the body, and to keep stress levels low.

Periodontal problems

Bacterial periodontitis has unfortunately become increasingly widespread in recent years. The periodontium, the tissue around the tooth which holds the tooth in the jawbone, becomes inflamed. The teeth are not in fact fused to the bone but are suspended within it by a group of tiny connective fibers known as the periodontal ligament. Periodontitis occurs not just when the gingiva (gum) is infected, but also when the deeper fibers are inflamed. This can lead to the destruction of the surrounding bone, causing the tooth to lose stability, start to come loose, and eventually even fall out.

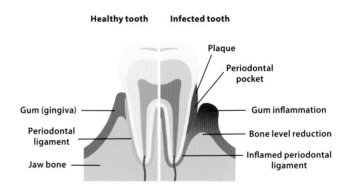

Unfortunately, periodontitis often has no symptoms and so can go unnoticed, making regular checks by a dentist all the more important. A laboratory can identify the bacteria found in gingival pockets while genetic predisposition can be investigated and fungal infection ruled out.

Depending on which bacteria are identified, dentists often prescribe high doses of antibiotics. In my experience (writes Jutta), you should think long and hard before using antibiotics. Consider if they are really necessary and how good the prognosis over the long term is. Prescribing antibiotics can sometimes make the situation worse in the long run. As dentists, we have questioned if we do enough (working in conjunction with a family doctor or alternative practitioner) to support a patient's healthy gut, aware as we are that oral mucosa (the mucous membrane lining the inside of the mouth) can often act as a mirror, reflecting the health of the intestinal mucosa.

Fortunately, alternative treatment with essential oils has been available for some time now. The oils are highly effective in supporting a healthy oral environment and can be applied by the patients themselves. The success of the therapy depends on targeted testing of the individual oils. This can be done using an aromatogram, a laboratory diagnostic technique in which swabs from between four and six gingival pockets are taken and are combined with the various oils in an agar culture medium. The effects of the individual oils on the bacteria soon become apparent and pinpoint those that can be used in treatment.

It is important to remember that infection caused by periodontitis bacteria is also always accompanied by dysbiosis, or "disrupted" sub-gingival bacterial flora, and a local infection that can vary in severity between individuals. This dysbiosis and the inflammation are mutually interdependent, and treatment is most successful when it addresses both the bacteria and the inflammation.

The advantage of using mouth rinses with essential oils is that you can both support your oral flora and deal with the inflammation. When used together with an aromatogram, it enables the dysbiotic bacteria environment in the gingival pocket to in effect be "reprogrammed" in a targeted way, bringing it back into symbiosis and soothing the inflammatory reaction. This is an important cornerstone of treatment for periodontitis, alongside regular preventive dental measures.

One advantage of using essential oils in oral health care is that they can be used over a longer period of time than antibiotics. And patients can also apply them themselves. Note that there should be regular breaks in treatment, however.

It is always rewarding when a patient finds that regular check-ups reveal a general improvement in their gum health. They might be so pleased with their progress and new sense of well-being that it gives them the impetus to make changes in other areas and even discover a new quality of life.

After brushing the teeth, add around 10 drops of the thyme or copaiba mixture to 1.4 fl oz (40 ml) of lukewarm water (see p. 70). Suck this through the teeth with some force for a couple of minutes to form an effective emulsion. The fluid that you then spit out should be whitish in color.

Now use an interdental brush to introduce some of the oil mixture into each of the spaces between your teeth. Massaging with the interdental brush reinforces the positive effects and a dentist can rinse the deep gingival pockets thoroughly.

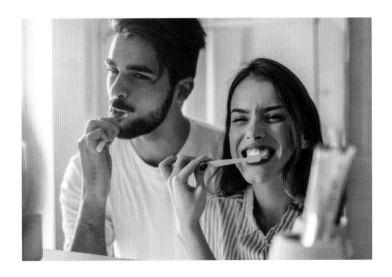

Tinctures of sage and calendula are particularly effective. However, do note that effectiveness may reduce with regular use, say after eight weeks, so it is best to alternate in order to prevent a reduction in effectiveness. Other essential oils that we have tested with success include manuka, niaouli, lemongrass, tea tree, red thyme, bay leaf, rosemary, cajeput, copaiba, and lemon.

While using a targeted mixture based on saliva testing to suit the individual is the most effective solution, the following are tried-and-tested:

Thyme mixture

5 drops of manuka essential oil
2 drops of copaiba essential oil
10 drops of lemongrass essential oil
10 drops of thyme essential oil
in 1 fl oz (30 ml) sesame oil

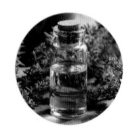

Copaiba mixture

8 drops of copaiba essential oil
2 drops of cinnamon essential oil
2 drops of eucalyptus essential oil
1 drop of frankincense essential oil
2 drops of lemon essential oil
in 1 fl oz (30 ml) sesame oil

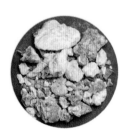

Oral candidiasis

You may be familiar with that unpleasant feeling when your skin is itchy and burning, or it feels tight, dry, and red, or flaky, or even when an open or weeping wound has formed, indicating the presence of a fungal infection. This can also occur in the mouth, but here, unfortunately, it often also goes unnoticed.

The most common oral pathogen is *Candida albicans* which, as the name suggests, is revealed by white spots on a reddish base inside the mouth, although they may only be noticeable under close inspection.

Candida is a pathogenic yeast that is particularly at home in the mucosa of the mouth, gut, or genitals. If you discover changes in your oral mucosa that make you suspect candida may be present, consult your doctor who will take a swab to be tested in a laboratory.

Candida does not generally only confine itself to the mouth; it may spread via the throat and stomach as far as the gut, and the reverse is just as likely to happen. For dentists, this means working closely with physicians and alternative practitioners with experience in this area. As candida infection (candidiasis) is not visible in the gut, close observation of the oral mucosa is important. If the infection becomes severe, the patient's entire immune system can be compromised.

Before treating candidiasis in the clinic, we first check whether the patient is suffering from heavy metal contamination, which can be caused by the presence of old amalgam tooth fillings. The candida fungus binds to heavy metals and multiplies when these are present. Therefore, if heavy metal contamination is detected in a patient, it makes sense to only offer treatment when it has been eliminated from the body and the source identified and dealt with.

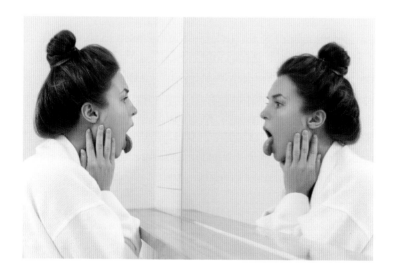

The textbook treatment for candidiasis is an antifungal medication, but in many cases this fails to address the cause of the infection. The natural balance of the cell environment may have been upset and weakened, while the level of lactic acid bacteria, for example, may be too low. The pH levels of the tissue may have skewed toward the acidic, harming the gut flora and leaving the door open for candida as a result. This is why serious illness is often accompanied by a fungal infection.

What can you do to get rid of these unwelcome guests and keep them at bay for as long as possible? A holistic approach starts primarily with nutrition and a deacidified diet. Candida loves sugar and isolated carbohydrates such as white flour, so you should eliminate these from your diet over a period of time.

Ask your family doctor or alternative practitioner to carry out a microbiological examination of a stool sample and try to build your good gut flora back up with probiotics. But alongside these measures, we also deploy essential oils as a secret weapon!

Treating Candida with oregano essential oil
Oregano oil is a powerful essential oil that has proved effective in tests against fungus as a result of its high phenol content. It is a particularly good choice to treat candida infection, as it soothes attendant symptoms such as flatulence and tiredness.

This oil has a very intense flavor that many patients find unpalatable, even when diluted with coconut oil. Taking it in capsule form is therefore a good alternative. It is important to drink plenty of water to assist the body's detoxification process. Studies have shown that oregano essential oil is highly effective against bacteria, viruses, and fungi, and it also prompts the release of many toxins and waste products, so the more you drink, the better you will tolerate the treatment.

The process of removing the destroyed microorganisms can be helped by taking a teaspoon of zeolite (no more than 1/5 oz or 6 g) once or twice a day. This is a powder of volcanic origin that has the effect of binding together and removing toxins.

The oregano oil/coconut oil mixture can also be applied topically to a fungal infection of the skin.

Do note, however, that oregano essential oil should **not** be consumed by women during pregnancy or when breastfeeding. Babies and children should also **not** be treated with oregano oil. It is a very powerful and effective natural remedy. Those taking oregano oil internally, who also suffer from an iron deficiency, should only take it two hours before or after meals, as it may inhibit iron intake.

If the oil makes your tongue or gums sting or burn, rinse your mouth with diluted tea tree oil. Any essential oil that boosts the immune system has the potential to help.

Mouth sensitivity

Unhealthy teeth and their associated problems can affect our physical well-being, just as the emotions can; the two are linked. And, in the same way, illness in the body can cause problems with the teeth and gums.

We are familiar with acupuncture meridians from Chinese medicine, which teaches that every tooth is linked to a particular meridian as well as to different organs and regions of the body. The incisors of the upper and lower jaw are related to the bladder and kidney meridian, for example. Therefore, when the bladder or kidney are affected by disease, these teeth should be checked for sources of inflammation. Similarly, hormonal change (such as during menopause or pregnancy) or infection in the abdomen can cause complaints that affect the incisors. An experienced dentist will also spot signs of other disease (HIV infection or bulimia, for example) in the mouth.

However, patients may not necessarily receive an "on the spot" diagnosis. This makes it important to build up a synergetic network with other therapists, including gut health therapists, dieticians, orthopedic experts, osteopaths, and physiotherapists, not to mention neurologists, alternative practitioners, psychologists, and holistic healers. Environmental medicine plays a pivotal role in dentistry as well, in particular in relation to the problems sometimes associated with the choice of materials used in crowns and fillings. No material is tolerated in the mouth as well as the natural tooth, which is why correct oral hygiene and regular dental checkups are so important, although it may sometimes seem as though dentists insist upon these at the risk of becoming annoying.

Hypersensitivity in the mouth is growing as a result of increasing environmental pressures, and an allergy test is often advisable. As a general rule, if you don't need to introduce anything into the mouth, it is best not to do so. Essential oils should therefore be used as a preventive measure.

Fortunately, there are a few tips that can see toothache sufferers through a weekend or a public holiday, or at least until the next available appointment at the clinic. It remains important to visit the dentist to establish what the problem is—dental caries (tooth decay), an exposed tooth neck, an infection, injury, or some other problem—so it can be treated appropriately. The oils can, of course, continue to be used as complementary treatments.

Toothaches

In an ideal world, everyone would be unfamiliar with the sensation of a tooth that is just beginning to hurt, or one that aches, throbs, or even hammers away in pain. You may try to disregard the pain at first, but eventually it becomes impossible to ignore. The following mixture of oils should bring some relief:

Isolated toothache

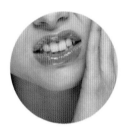

1 drop of cajeput essential oil
10 drops of clove essential oil
1 drop of thyme essential oil
1 drop of bay leaf essential oil
1 drop of niaouli essential oil
in 1 fl oz (30 ml) sesame oil

Apply the mixture to a cotton bud and swab the tooth and surrounding gum. Alternatively, dampen a cotton pad or piece of gauze with the mixture and hold it within the cheek pocket against the affected area.

The flavor is very intense and not to everyone's liking, but the results are generally very good.

Teething problems in infants

The first challenge in a young baby's life is when the milk teeth start to emerge. These first tiny teeth generally appear at about six months, with a full set of milk teeth (a total of twenty) generally forming by the thirtieth month. The time at which the teeth first start emerging varies greatly between children; some even have teeth at birth, while others wait months.

Increased saliva flow and fussiness in children are signs that their teeth are starting to erupt. They will be cranky, often suffering from diarrhea or stomach cramps, and they tend to cry a lot, disturbing everyone's sleep.

Lavender or mandarin essential oil in a room diffuser will help to relax a baby and the parents (or carers). A diffuser is a device in which essential oils are mixed with water and nebulized to fragrance the air in a room. It will promote a greater sense of security and calm in a baby. Try to reduce external stimuli too. As the gut is also affected, you can start to give gentle abdominal massage.

Slight teething

2 drops of Roman chamomile essential oil
4 drops of lavender essential oil
2 drops of clove essential oil
in a mixture of ½ fl oz (15 ml) St John's
wort oil and 15 ml sesame oil

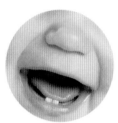

Gentle teething

1 drop of frankincense essential oil
1 drop of rose essential oil
1 drop of Roman chamomile essential oil
1 drop of lavender essential oil
1 drop of ylang-ylang essential oil
1 drop of mandarin essential oil
in a mixture of ½ fl oz (15 ml) St John's wort oil and ½ fl oz
(15 ml) jojoba oil

These oil mixtures can be applied topically to the cheeks. They
are relaxing and bring a sense of security.

At the age of six months, a baby's feet can also be massaged
with lavender. Calm your child by treating the foot pressure
points, the tips of the toes, and the areas between them.

Applying gentle pressure on the jaw also reduces the pain.
Give the baby iris root to chew, its properties should also help
to calm the baby. Boil the roots regularly to keep them hygienic
or the carbohydrates contained in the roots could become a
breeding ground for bacteria.

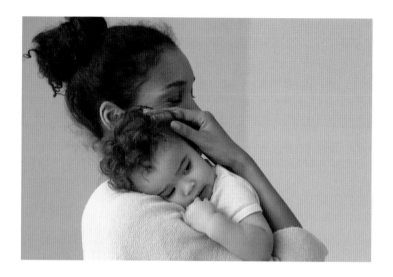

Plenty of physical contact and rhythmic movements while holding and carrying a baby can also help.

Do note that using essential oils for newborns and babies under the age of six months is **not** recommended, as they are still very sensitive to smells at this age. The one exception here is frankincense oil, which should always be diluted with a carrier oil (see below).

It was used in ancient times to mitigate the stress of birth for newborns, with the oil being gently massaged into their heads. It is no coincidence that the infant Jesus was brought frankincense by the Three Wise Men.

A drop of Roman chamomile can be mixed with a tablespoon of coconut oil and gently rubbed into the area of painful gum, but don't force it if the child doesn't like the taste. If a baby is being given homeopathic remedies, wait for a while before using chamomile in order not to disrupt their effects.

Chamomile can also be taken as a tea or added to a bath. For the latter, mix one drop of Roman chamomile oil with a tablespoon of sea salt and a teaspoon of carrier oil, and pour the mixture into the baby's bathwater.

Unfortunately, increased saliva production during teething often reddens the soft skin of a baby's lips and face, which can then become inflamed. The following soothing combination will help to protect the skin from moisture and keep it rosy.

Baby skincare
1 tablespoon shea butter
1 drop of lavender essential oil

Store in a glass jar and only use a tiny amount, rubbed in gently with the fingertip as required.

It is important to remember that dental caries and gingivitis are infectious diseases, hence the need for parents to optimize their own oral hygiene and use the oils recommended in order not to infect their baby (see also 'One request' p. 41).

As a rule, essential oils should only be used for children in diluted form, with just one drop of essential oil in one table-spoon of carrier oil. For babies under the age of 6 months, essential oils are ***not*** recommended, the one exception being frankincense (see p. 81).

For infants aged 6 months to 3 years, the following essential oils mentioned in this book are suitable: Roman chamomile, rose, orange, mandarin, copaiba, lavender, and frankincense. All other oils mentioned in this book are not recommended for this age group, especially eucalyptus oil, which can be harmful to small children because of its strongly mucolytic (loosens mucus) effect.

For children aged 3 years and above, all essential oils from this book can be used ***except*** the following: peppermint, cinnamon, clove (can be used in mixtures but not for single use), oregano. However, the latter (peppermint, cinnamon, clove, oregano) are suitable for school children, aged 6 and above.

Rosemary should not be used for children under the age of 4.

Make sure you use only high-quality natural essential oils.

Wisdom teeth

Milk teeth are not the only teeth that can cause problems when they begin to emerge; wisdom teeth may also be troublesome in later life. Pericoronitis can occur when the jaw is too small to accommodate the teeth. The wisdom teeth may only emerge halfway and remain partly covered by mucosa. Food and bacteria can then collect under this "hood," and, if the immune system is weakened or significant pressure or emotional stress are involved, infection and inflammation can soon set in.

Opening the mouth wide can become difficult, but essential oils should help. An appointment with a dentist should be made as soon as possible, however. Inflammation of this kind must be taken seriously because it can quickly spread into deeper areas via the soft tissue of the tooth neck and requires the attention of a dental expert to determine the next step.

In my clinic, we clean the pockets carefully, rinse them with our oil mixtures, and apply a tamponade with an oil paste for at least thirty minutes.

Wisdom tooth pain relief

3 drops of eucalyptus essential oil
4 drops of tea tree essential oil
6 drops of clove essential oil
1 drop of Ravensara essential oil
4 drops of thyme essential oil
4 drops of lemongrass essential oil
2 drops of essential rosemary oil
in 1 fl oz (30 ml) sesame oil

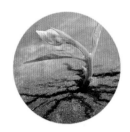

Apply this mixture carefully with a cotton bud or use it combined with water as a mouth rinse.

According to the Chinese theory of meridians, the wisdom teeth are connected to the heart, small intestine, and the triple warmer meridian, among others. It could therefore be helpful to consider the following:

In general, the heart meridian represents love, joy in life, communication, enthusiasm, calm, and deep sleep. It reacts positively to frankincense, neroli, orange blossom, and sandalwood oil. The small intestine meridian is connected with energy flow, anxiety, and the inner center, and normally relieves the heart from the pressures of everyday trivialities and concerns. It can be boosted with the scent of spikenard and bergamot. Spikenard is, unfortunately, an endangered plant species and cannot be harvested in the wild for sale, although the essential oil may become available once again from farmed sources in the future. In the meantime, however, bergamot essential oil can be of help. The triple warmer meridian cannot be directly associated with any specific organ but regulates the acquisition and distribution of physical energy. Marjoram, lemon balm, and rose oil have proved effective in treating it.

Meridian-boosting oils can be mixed with a carrier oil and applied externally for support on an emotional level when having problems with wisdom teeth in general. Apply a few drops of your personal mixture (depending on the theme(s) that you think apply in your particular case), or the mixture we suggest below, to a flannel wash mitt and place it against your cheek. If you need a cooling effect, you might want to place a few ice cubes or a cold pack inside the mitt. Be careful not to make your cheeks too cold. It is best to remove the cooling pack after a few minutes (always stop if your cheeks or jaw start to feel numb), pause, and then apply again.

Soul sustenance
2 drops of frankincense essential oil
2 drops of osmanthus essential oil
2 drops of spruce essential oil
2 drops of lavender essential oil
2 drops of cedarwood essential oil
5 drops of grapefruit essential oil
10 drops of sandalwood essential oil
in 1 fl oz (30 ml) sesame oil

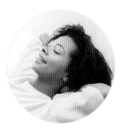

Mouth ulcers

Mouth ulcers are small, round cankerous formations with a white base that develop in and around mucous membranes. The exact cause of mouth ulcers is yet to be determined, but experts assume that several factors can trigger them, ranging from a virus or food intolerance to a person's emotional state. Hormonal factors may also be involved. Constant irritation of the gum, by a retainer, for example, may increase the chances of mouth ulcers developing, and stress or a weakened immune system are also possible causes. Vitamin B12, iron, or folic acid deficiency appear to result in the cumulative formation of mouth ulcers, in which case a blood test to investigate the patient's nutritional state can be a good way forward.

Everyone is susceptible to mouth ulcers at some point. They seem to occur at random, causing sudden and sharp pain, accompanied by an itching or burning sensation in the affected area. They are especially painful when eating, swallowing, or speaking. The degree of pain is not affected by the size of the mouth ulcer but by its location, and ulcers on the tongue are particularly unpleasant.

Mouth ulcers generally heal by themselves after eight to ten days, but the application of tea tree oil can help to speed things up. Some people use a cotton bud to dab it onto the ulcers neat, while others prefer to dilute it.

Cold sores

Unlike mouth ulcers, the herpes virus infection occurs very rarely in mucous membranes, but instead is generally located on the exterior of the lips. Herpes sores, otherwise known as "cold sores," are a symptom of the herpes simplex virus, which causes a frequently recurring infection.

In a typical case, tingling blisters with a reddened base appear, in which pus forms after two or three days. The blisters burst and weep and are highly infectious during this phase. A hard crust will then form and heal, fortunately without leaving a scar in most cases.

Initial infection with herpes is through smear infection, and the virus then lives on in the nerve cells of the affected person for the rest of their life. When it recurs, the virus migrates from the nerve cells down nerve pathways to the skin, where it causes the typical symptoms.

The actual cause of recurrences is the source of much speculation and research, but likely candidates include feverish infection, UV light exposure, excessive heat or cold, situations causing mental or physical stress, local trauma, or hormonal change.

As increasing resistance builds against traditional textbook herpes remedies, we can take advantage of the many different properties of essential oils. Applying an oil with dab on the lips at the first sign of the tingling sensation is very important. Habitual sufferers will instantly recognize the early symptoms of a flare-up. Lavender oil can be applied neat with a cotton bud several times a day and has proved its worth; it doesn't burn when applied and has a pleasant fragrance. Tea tree, manuka, and peppermint oil are also effective, although they should be diluted with a carrier oil.

Lemon balm oil has proved particularly effective in the clinic, and we have noted that regular use reduces the frequency of cold sores. It is one of the most expensive oils, which might seem odd to anyone with experience of growing lemon balm in their garden, knowing how quickly it spreads. Extracting the essential oil is difficult, however, and if conditions are not quite right during growth and harvest, almost no essential oil is obtained through distillation.

Make use of any of the oils that boost the immune system. Clove, oregano, thyme, lemongrass, rosemary, lemon, peppermint, or cinnamon essential oil are all suitable for application to the reflex zones of the feet, either as individual oils or as part of a mixture.

Alkaline baths to which lavender or eucalyptus oil has been added are also very good at boosting the body's defenses. Take a handful of sea salt, 5 drops of the essential oil, and a dash of carrier oil, mix together, and add the mixture to the bathwater.

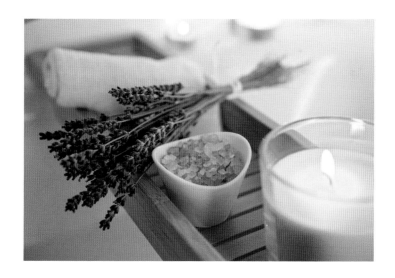

Dry mouth

The action of spitting conveys anger or frustration, but being unable to produce enough saliva to spit is equally unpleasant from a clinical perspective. A dry mouth, also known as xerostomia, may have a wide variety of causes.

It can arise as a side effect of medications such as painkillers, antibiotics, or psychotherapeutic drugs, or as a result of radiotherapy and/or chemotherapy. Hormonal changes during pregnancy or breastfeeding may also be a cause, and smoking, drinking alcohol, and excessive stress can lead to a dry mouth. As people age, they tend to drink less liquid and become dehydrated. Those who sleep with their mouths open, or indeed snore, will also lose moisture. Dry mouth is also an indicator of as yet undiagnosed disease such as diabetes or thyroid malfunction.

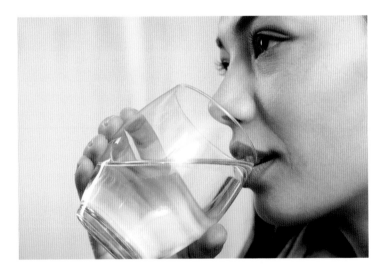

Being unable to spit in the literal sense is because the saliva has become viscous and tacky. The tongue feels raw and swollen and seems to stick to the palate. The sense of taste is impaired, and it can be difficult to swallow or speak. The teeth are more sensitive to temperature, resulting in unpleasant mouth odor. Gums are more susceptible to inflammation, and dentures that normally fit well can suddenly cause problems.

The moisturizing properties of saliva help to protect our teeth and gums; it neutralizes acids, while the calcium and phosphates dissolved in spit naturally remineralize the enamel.

If the ability to produce saliva becomes impaired, long-term results include heightened susceptibility to dental caries and a tendency to develop gingivitis, so it is important to identify the causes and to initiate treatment where appropriate.

One step that can be taken straight away is to adopt what is known as a "chewing diet." Intensive chewing movements activate the muscles of the mouth and tongue, stimulating the salivary glands to increase production. It can also help to chew sugar-free, xylitol chewing gum between meals. Sage, chamomile, or ginger tea can also often bring relief.

Increased saliva flow

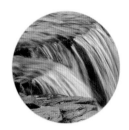

1 drop of sage essential oil
2 drops of clove essential oil
10 drops of lemon essential oil
15 drops of orange essential oil
2 drops of fennel essential oil
2 drops of ginger essential oil
in 1 fl oz (30 ml) sesame oil

Fill a pipette with the above mixture and squeeze it into your mouth. Rinse for around two minutes, before spitting it out or swallowing it.

Tooth decay

The term dental caries describes tooth decay caused by the metabolic processes of bacteria. It has evolved into a typical lifestyle disease of the modern era. Oral bacteria need sugar for their metabolism. This is provided by our diet, particularly by foods and drinks that are sweet or rich in carbohydrates and cause a thick film of bacteria known as plaque to form on the surface of the enamel and in the spaces between the teeth. If this remains in place over the long term, lactic acids are produced through bacterial metabolism. These acids demineralize the enamel by releasing calcium ions and the enamel becomes porous. This allows microorganisms to enter the tooth and destroy it from within.

One of the functions of saliva, which is enhanced with minerals, is to harden tooth enamel, although it finds it hard to keep up with constant snacking between meals and sweetened drinks.

People are susceptible to dental caries to different degrees. Levels of acid in the saliva vary between individuals—the lower the pH value, the more intense the acid attack on the teeth.

Prevention, oral care, and diet help to combat the development of dental caries.

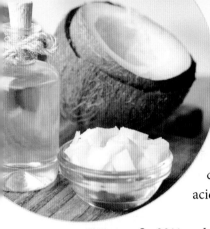

Coconut oil for a healthy, tooth-friendly diet

Coconut oil has natural antibacterial and anti-inflammatory properties that can be used to promote dental health. It has a high content of lauric acid, a medium-chain fatty acid capable of dissolving bacterial cell walls.

In 2011 and 2012, the Athlone Institute of Technolgy in Ireland conducted a study identifying a link between coconut oil and dental caries. The study used untreated oil alongside oil that had been exposed to a digestive enzyme. The "pre-digested" variant turned out to be a natural antibiotic against most strains of *Streptococcus*, the main pathogen that causes dental caries. It was equally effective in combating a particular yeast that is considered the second-most powerful cause. Even small amounts of the oil proved highly effective, and Dr Damien Brady, who led the study, views enzyme-modified coconut oil as a viable alternative to conventional dental care products. The study has attracted heavy criticism, however, and doubts have been expressed about the enzyme pretreatment of the coconut oil in particular. In an Indian study on combating dental caries published in 2016, the scientific team compared the use of chlorhexidine and coconut oil (that had not been altered with an enzyme) in oral care for school-age children. In both groups, it proved possible to contain the bacteria causing caries within thirty days.

As oral care products with coconut oil are scarce (writes Jutta), I recommend using coconut oil for oil pulling. This also has a positive effect on mouth flora.

Coconut oil can be used without any essential oils, whereas it is recommended to use sesame oil as a carrier oil when using essential oils (see p. 18).

Oil pulling

Daily oil pulling is a traditional Ayurvedic treatment. The coconut oil immediately liquefies in the mouth and slowly mixes with the saliva. It can be rinsed around the teeth and should penetrate into the gaps between them to be fully effective. Bacteria that have accumulated here are destroyed, and the mouth is cleansed of harmful substances.

Perform the oil pulling treatment every morning first thing and on an empty stomach (before breakfast).

Hold approximately one tablespoon of coconut oil in your mouth and roll it around your tongue, pulling and sucking it through the gaps between your teeth. Do this for at least six minutes (some suggest up to twenty minutes).

Spit out and flush away the mixture when you have finished (avoid swallowing it). Rinse out your mouth with water and enjoy breakfast. Wait half an hour before cleaning your teeth thoroughly.

In 2015 a clinical study was carried out at Kannur Dental College in Kerala, India, investigating in part whether coconut oil was suitable for treating gingivitis. Gargling or rinsing the mouth with oil is a tried-and-true treatment for all kinds of inflammations, but the aim in this case was to discover in a scientific way exactly how effective it might be. Sesame and sunflower oils are thought to be effective treatments of gingivitis caused by plaque, but this study is the first to examine the use of coconut oil for such a purpose. The composition of coconut oil is unique: up to 50 percent of its mostly medium-chain fatty acids are made up of lauric acid, which has powerful anti-inflammatory and antibiotic properties. The use of coconut oil caused a significant reduction in plaque and gingivitis, and a clear improvement in symptoms was visible from as early as the seventh day of application.

Both Jutta and Karin recommend adding a few drops of copaiba oil to the coconut oil to enhance its effects still further.

Copaiba *(Copaifera reticulata)*

Botanical family: *Fabaceae* (legumes)
Copaiba essential oil is obtained
through steam distillation of gum resin.

The gumlike resin copaiba is found in
a variety of both evergreen and decid-
uous trees growing in South America
and Asia that are known collectively
as the copal tree. Copal trees are hardy
and adaptable and grow in wetlands and
forests. They reach a height of up to 130 ft
(40 m) and living for up to 400 years. To reach
the coveted gum, a small hole is bored in the trunk
and the resulting liquid diverted into a container, in much the
same way as maple syrup is collected. A tree can be tapped in
this way two or three times a year, producing up to a gallon
(4–5 liters) of copaiba on average. To protect the tree from fungus and pests, the hole is stopped up with clay after tapping.

The Aztecs used copaiba gum as frankincense and the word
copelli approximates to smoke in their language. The *curanderos,*
the local healers and shamans of Brazil, used copaiba to
drive away negative energy and soothe pain and inflammation.
The gum is also very kind to the skin and helps wounds to
heal. My family and I (writes Karin) had a very good outcome
with it when we treated our dog's wound after it was bitten by
another dog.

I like to call copaiba "copycat oil" because it can enhance the effects of another oil; peppermint oil has a similar property, but it has a strong fragrance of its own. Copaiba oil has a subtle, gently balsamic scent and mixes very well with blossom oils, which can be expensive.

Always make sure you buy 100 percent pure copaiba oil. Some retailers reduce its price by diluting it.

Rinsing the mouth with coconut oil mixed with copaiba oil can actually be a pleasant experience. It has a mild taste of its own, whereas other essential oils recommended as additives for mouthwash are more intense, with distinctive flavors and fragrances.

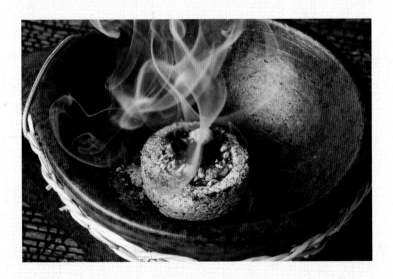

Copaiba can also be used in mouthwashes due to its high levels of beta-caryophyllene, which studies have shown to be effective against inflammation. It also helps to combat bacteria and fungi.

Copaiba strengthens the entire body and promotes the natural function of numerous organs.

Bad breath

Most of us have experienced the anxiety caused by a fear of bad breath. We worry about speaking to or standing too close to someone else, whether at work, at home, or out and about. Almost half of us think that our breath smells.

Fortunately, this is often not the case, and only about 25 percent of people actually suffer from occasional bad breath, also known as halitosis. Only around 10 percent of the population suffers from chronic mouth odor.

Fear of bad breath can turn into a real phobia. Bad breath is not dangerous, of course, but anxiety about it can lead to excessive use of mouthwashes or chewing gum, and, in particularly extreme cases, to the avoidance of close human contact. Sufferers constantly check their breath and become increasingly insecure.

We offer patients special halitosis advice clinics (writes Jutta) in which we examine the breath and investigate possible causes, take a general medical history, identify current medication, establish levels of water intake and whether someone snores or has misaligned teeth.

The effects of garlic, alcohol, and nicotine are temporary and will not cause lasting problems. What we are talking about here is actual bad breath that requires closer investigation.

You would be forgiven for thinking that the causes of bad breath lie in the stomach, but this is not necessarily the case. In fact, the most common cause of unpleasant odor is a concentration of bacteria in the mouth, and, in nine out of ten cases, bad breath arises within the mouth cavity. This is where you can take action yourself.

These generally anaerobic (able to survive without oxygen) bacteria are located between the teeth, in the gingival pockets, or in decaying teeth. They are also mostly found on the tongue, however, with the rear third of this muscle being particularly affected. The ridges and valleys of the back of the tongue are ideal places for the bacteria to collect. This is where bacteria transform leftover food particles, especially from protein-rich food, into hydrosulfides that can smell like rotten eggs or even into cadaverine, a by-product of decomposition. The results can be very noticeable.

There is normally a healthy equilibrium between aerobic bacteria and those that cause decay. However, if the balance is upset, perhaps by eating a particular diet or food that is too acidic, by drinking too much alcohol or coffee, or indeed by taking in insufficient fluids, then this harmony can be disrupted over the long term. A thick coating of a whitish, yellowish, or even brown color may then be seen on the tongue.

The solution is fairly simple and involves brushing not just the teeth, but also the back of the tongue, a practice that has been common in Asia for many hundreds of years. Clinical studies have proven the effect of this tried-and-true technique.

As part of a home dental care regime, try to use an additional tongue brush or scraper once a day (plastic or metal). Drag it across the tongue several times from the back to the front. Stick your tongue out as far as possible as you do so, even gently gripping it with one hand. Any slight gag reflex will settle over time.

For even more impressive results, add a couple of drops of our special mixture of essential oils on your tongue.

Breath freshener

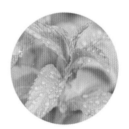

15 drops of myrtle essential oil
3 drops of rosemary essential oil
3 drops of copaiba essential oil
3 drops of sage essential oil
5 drops of spearmint essential oil
5 drops of thyme essential oil
in 1 fl oz (30 ml) sesame oil

Myrtle *(Myrtus communis)*

Botanical family:
Myrtaceae (myrtle family)

Myrtle essential oil is obtained through steam distillation of the leaves.

The evergreen myrtle bush is common in North Africa, especially in Tunisia and Morocco. It grows to a height of up to 15 ft (5 m) and forms small white flowers from May to August.

The essential oil has a generally cleansing effect on the body and can help to break up mucus. It promotes healthy mouth flora when used in a mouthwash, and will also harmonize the thyroid gland and ovaries, as discovered by the French practitioner, educator, and author Dr Daniel Pénoël, one of the pioneers of the therapeutic uses of essential oils.

Rosemary *(Rosmarinus officinalis)*
Botanical family:
Lamiaceae (labiates)
Rosemary essential oil is obtained
through steam distillation of
the leaves.

This evergreen plant loves a warm,
dry climate and is a very popular herb,
particularly in Mediterranean cuisine.
It is also used in naturopathic treatments.

Just like oregano and thyme, rosemary also has
powerful cleansing properties—the air in hospitals in
France was cleansed and freshened with the scent of rosemary
until the 1920s. The essential oil can be used for gargling when
mixed with water or a carrier oil. It is good for the throat and
boosts the liver.

Do note that rosemary should **not** be used for children under
the age of four, or by anyone who is taking medication for high
blood pressure.

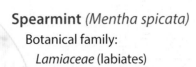

Spearmint *(Mentha spicata)*

Botanical family:
Lamiaceae (labiates)

Spearmint essential oil is obtained through steam distillation of the leaves.

We all remember the smell of spearmint from our childhood (or perhaps adult) chewing gum years. Just a single drop of this essential oil in a mouthwash can help to deliver a wonderfully fresh feeling in the mouth.

Spearmint essential oil also stimulates the metabolism, while its scent brings a sense of balance and harmony.

Thyme *(Thymus vulgaris)*
Botanical family:
Lamiaceae (labiates)
Thyme essential oil is obtained
through steam distillation of the
leaves, blossom, and stems.

Thyme is one of the most powerful herbs and was widely used by the ancients, who left us with precise descriptions of their use in old documents.

Thyme is much prized in oral hygiene due to its powerful cleansing properties. It can also provide a holistic boost when you feel exhausted and drained.

Do note that if you are sensitive, inhaling the essential oil directly from the bottle can irritate the nasal mucous membranes. Use it in a carrier oil to avoid any soreness.

Stress and teeth

There are times in life when we feel particularly tired and stressed, which can also have an impact on our teeth.

For many people, their experience of long-term stress, bound up with high expectations and pressurized situations, occurs in particular at work, which is then compounded by worries and concern about the future. Advances in technology and digitization mean that the professional world is constantly changing and developing. Workers find themselves needing to be enormously flexible in order to adapt to new circumstances, and of course anxieties and emergencies at home and in family life may also be involved.

What effect does this have on us physically? Stress produces acids and the body then tries to protect its internal organs against attack by extracting alkaline substances (to neutralize the acid) from mineral deposits in the teeth, bones, and scalp, for example.

This tension is often unconsciously incorporated into our sleep and processed through teeth-grinding (bruxism). Grinding, pressing, or chattering the teeth with significant force places a huge burden on the teeth and jaws. Certain essential oils can help with this by inducing relaxation and reducing stress before sleep. Frankincense, lavender, cedarwood, vetiver, orange, and mandarin oil are particularly soothing. They can either be nebulized individually in an ultrasound diffuser in the bedroom or combined to produce a mixture of oils that can be used in a relaxing, calming foot massage. Ask your partner to spoil you with a stress-reducing massage.

If an anti-stress combination of oils can "bring you down" from excessively high stress levels during the day, it may be worth considering just what is causing the stress in the first place. In the meantime, however, essential oils can certainly soothe the soul during relatively short bouts of emotional upset or physical challenges.

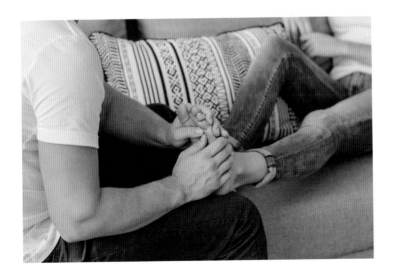

Essential oil "stars"

An essential oil in its purest form is always particularly special (writes Karin), although the process of obtaining the oil from certain plants can be laborious or require considerable amounts of plant matter, making the essential oil expensive. It is important not to waste any part of the plant, by accelerating the distillation process, for example. An essential oil should also contain all its active ingredients.

The following pages contain several examples of these exclusive essential oil "stars," oils that are extremely valuable and versatile but also prima donnas in how difficult they are to produce.

Rose *(Rosa damascena)*
Botanical family:
Rosaceae (rose family)
Rose essential oil is obtained through steam distillation of the flowers.

Roses contain around 400 active ingredients. The essential oil is certainly one of the most expensive, which is not surprising when you learn that 8,820–11,000 lb (4–5,000 kg) of fresh blooms are required to make just over 2 lb (1 kg) of rose essential oil—making it almost worth its weight in gold!

A distinction is drawn between essential oils derived from the Bulgarian rose and those from the Moroccan rose, whose different compositions deliver very different effects.

The first person to distill rose oil was the Persian physician, scholar, and philosopher Avicenna (Arabic: Ibn Sina, 980–1037CE), who also made use of the rose water that was a by-product. He wrote a detailed work dedicated to the therapeutic uses of the rose, and it is surprising to discover just how accurate his observations were back then. The Damask rose is now principally grown in Bulgaria, although its name hints at its origins in Damascus, Syria. It was probably Crusaders returning from the East who first introduced it to Europe in the 12th century.

The flowers are harvested in the early hours of the morning before sunrise, when their essential oil content is at its highest. The content declines during the day, reducing the potential yield. Distillation must be carried out speedily as the leaves start to ferment if stored for any length of time. Attending the rose harvest in the so-called Rose Valley in Bulgaria is a dream that I hope to realize one day.

With its pleasant connotations, the concept of rose oil speaks to many strongly on an emotional level. For some, however, its scent is overpowering, and some people even go so far as to dislike it, perhaps because it is linked to some deep emotional trauma through its associations with a past event. One therapy in Ayurveda uses essential oils to identify a client's psychological issues, a technique I was introduced to by Ayurvedic and alternative health practitioner and author Erika Diehl. It involves the client smelling various scents, with their eyes closed, while the therapist observes the way they react with their body language and posture. Any "conflict oils" (I call them "stink oils") discovered during the therapy will then correlate with the challenges that the client should address more closely in order to reestablish equilibrium. Rose oil is associated with a person's feminine side, with their relationship with their mother, for example, or with women in general. A person who was separated from their mother directly after birth may consequently find the scent of roses problematic.

German alternative practitioner in psychotherapy Tamara Mauerberger explains how such traumatic birth experiences can be balanced out with a healing rose bath in which mother and baby bathe together in water mixed with rose oil (one drop of rose oil to one cup of sea salt added to the bathwater). The still-wet baby is then laid on the naked torso of the mother and both are wrapped in towels and blankets. This helps to create a feeling of connection after the birth.

There is no substitute for the scent of rose oil and its associations with feelings of unconditional love and acceptance, hence it is a great asset in forging strong mother–child relationships and in romantic partnerships.

Rose essential oil can also be used in a number of different ways on a physical level: it strengthens tissue, reduces the formation of scars, mitigates inflammatory processes, delivers relaxation, and helps to deal with anxiety. It also has a harmonizing and balancing effect, lifting the spirits and calming the mind.

Rose oil can soothe feelings of vulnerability, which is why it is also included in the mixture recommended for teething infants (see p. 79).

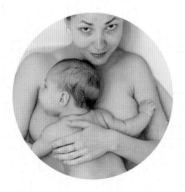

Lemon balm *(Melissa officinalis)*
Botanical family:
Lamiaceae (labiates)
Lemon balm essential oil is obtained from the leaves and stems before the plant flowers.

As mentioned earlier, the lemon balm plant grows vigorously, but it can be a bit of a diva as far as its essential oil is concerned, hence costing only just a little less than rose oil. I read a report of how after two male harvest workers had been yelling at one another across a field of lemon balm, the subsequent oil yield from that field was very low. To test the apparent effect of having submitted the plants to the shouting workers, the owner instead asked female workers to call out compliments to one another across a similar field. The plants exposed to the female workers went on to yield above average amounts of essential oil.

Such results will come as no surprise to followers of the findings published by Japanese researcher and author Masuro Emoto (1943–2014), who discovered that words exert an influence on water. If you say a word like "love" to a sample of water, or play classical music in its vicinity, it will form beautiful harmonious ice crystals when frozen, whereas abusive language will result in ugly, asymmetrical patterns. Since plants are living organisms, they react to vibrations, including the vibrations of speech.

Lemon balm essential oil deserves special mention for its use in the treatment of herpes infections. It also calms the mind and lifts the spirits.

Sandalwood *(Santalum album)*
Botanical family:
Santalaceae (sandalwood family)
Sandalwood essential oil is obtained through steam distillation of the wood.

Sandalwood is a particularly rare essential oil, not because of the small yield that the sandalwood tree produces, but rather because of the length of time that must expire before it is harvested. The oil yielded by this partially parasitic tree, which requires a host tree to survive, improves with the age of the tree. Until a couple of years ago, a sandalwood tree would not be harvested until it was forty years old, at which point it could yield up to 440 lb (200 kg) of essential oil. Sandalwood is highly prized, however, as it is also used for religious purposes, in incense sticks and in holy shrines and carvings. As a result, there has been much illegal felling of the tree, which means that it is now threatened with extinction and is a protected species. Every sandalwood tree in India is registered and remains the property of the state, even if it is located on private land.

An alternative is *Santalum paniculatum*, the sandalwood grown in Hawaii, which is sustainably farmed as a cultivated species. It has the same calming, uplifting, and reassuring effects, hence the inclusion of this special essential oil as an ingredient in the soul sustenance mixture (see p. 85).

However, essential oils in their purest form do not have to be expensive. Examples include the essential oils we use in our own mixtures. They are very versatile and yet affordable, such as lemon, orange, cedarwood, lemongrass, myrtle, and spearmint oil. These will be highly effective without breaking the bank.

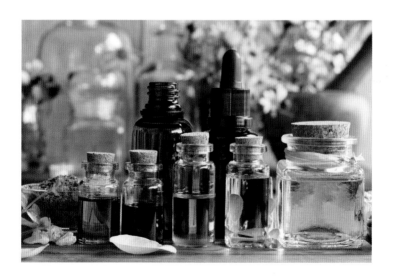

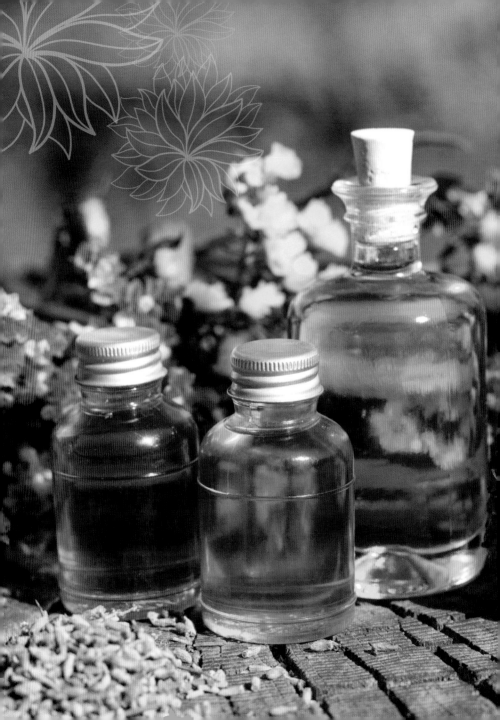

Epilogue

We have our adult teeth for life. They might be a source of torment when they first emerge, sometimes cause problems once they have arrived, and are just as troublesome when they finally have to go. So we wish you the best dental health always, with gleaming white teeth that are healthy and robust. We hope our tips will help you to achieve this.

We have explained a number of gentle ways in which to work with essential oils to support your own dental health and oral hygiene, and hopefully you will be more relaxed the next time you visit the dentist. After your appointment, you might even hear yourself saying, "Great! I wasn't anxious at all and there was no need for the drill!"

We would like to give our sincere thanks to Maria Kageaki, Caroline Adelskamp, Martina Kirchmayer, Lieselotte Büchler, and Irene Kessler, who stood by us like midwives during the last "push" in this book's creation.

We would also like to thank Florian Beier from the photography studio Marek & Beier in Munich for the wonderful photos from the dental clinic.

With all good wishes
Jutta Schreiber, D.M.D., and Karin Opitz-Kreher

Recommended reading

Fischer-Rizzi, Susanne: *Complete Aromatherapy Handbook: Essential Oils for Radiant Health*, Sterling Publishing Co. 1991

Hirschi, Gertrud: *Mudras, Yoga in your Hands*, Red Wheel/Weiser, 2000

Life Science Publishing (Hrsg): *Essential Oils Pocket Reference* (8th edition), Life Science Publishing, Lehi (Utah, USA) 2019

Price, Shirley: *Aromatherapy for Common Ailments* (Gaia Series), Fireside, 1991

Schrott, Ernst: *Marma Therapy: The Healing Power of Ayurvedic Vital Point Massage*, Singing Dragon, 2015

Tisserand, Robert: *The Art of Aromatherapy: The Healing and Beautifying Properties of the Essential Oils of Flowers and Herbs*, Healing Arts Press, 1978

Worwood, Valerie Ann: *The Fragrant Mind – Aromatherapy for Personality, Mind, Mood and Emotion*, Bantam Books/Transworld, London 1997

Picture credits

About the authors

Jutta Schreiber, D.M.D., has been working as a dentist for more than thirty years, specializing in holistic and naturopathic approaches at her own clinic in Neubiberg, Germany. Her methodology includes materials testing and exclusion, identifying interference zones, homeopathy, anthroposophical techniques, bioresonance, matrix rhythm therapy, and much more. She has also been using essential oils successfully in her clinic for many years. Since 2022 Jutta has worked with various dental practices as a consultant on dental and oral health, applying her knowledge and expertise in the field of essential oils.

Karin Opitz-Kreher has qualifications in aura soma, aura soma bodywork, and foot reflex zone reharmonization. She works in her own wellness clinic, specializing in stress reduction and harmonization. Karin has been making use of traditional knowledge of essential oils and passing this on to others in workshops since 2013.

Powerful yet concise, this revolutionary guide summarizes the Hawaiian ritual of forgiveness and offers methods for immediately creating positive effects in everyday life. Ho'oponopono consists of four consequent magic sentences: "I am sorry. Please forgive me. I love you. Thank you." By addressing issues using these simple sentences we get to own our feelings, and accept unconditional love, so that unhealthy situations transform into favorable experiences.

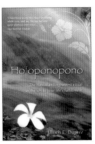

Ulrich Emil Duprée
Ho'oponopono
The Hawaiian forgiveness ritual as the key to your life's fulfillment
Paperback, full-color throughout, 96 pages
ISBN 978-1-84409-597-1

Healing Crystals is a comprehensive and up-to-date directory of 555 healing gemstones, presented in a practical and handy pocket guide format. In the revised edition of his bestseller, Michael Gienger, famous for his pioneering work in the field of crystal healing, describes the characteristics and healing powers of each crystal in a clear, concise, and precise style, accompanied by four-color photographs.

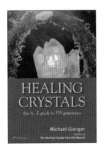

Michael Gienger
Healing Crystals
the A–Z guide to 555 gemstones, 2nd edition
Paperback, full-color throughout, 128 pages
ISBN 978-1-84409-647-3

Drawing on the Huna Hawaiian shamanic tradition as well as other shamanic and energetic practices and rituals, the authors show how to connect with our Aumakua, which includes our close relatives, ancestors stretching back thousands of years, and our spiritual ancestors or karmic family, for healing and self-development.

Jeanne Ruland & Shantidevi
Ancestral Healing for Your Spiritual and Genetic Families
Understanding Our Energy Cycles for Health and Healing
Paperback, full-color throughout, 112 pages
ISBN 978-1-64411-034-8

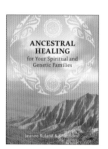

In this full-color pocket guide featuring beautiful animal photos, the authors introduce 45 important spirit animals alphabetically and explore their wisdom. They provide a meditative journey to help you discover which animal is your personal soul companion and offer practices to intuitively find the right power animal for a given situation.

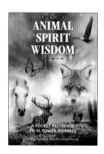

Phillip Kansa, Elke Kirchner-Young
Animal Spirit Wisdom
A Pocket Reference to 45 Power Animals
Paperback, full-color throughout, 112 pages
ISBN 978-1-64411-115-4

There is more than one type of angel, not just those with wings. For thousands of years, people seeking advice or wanting to give thanks to nature have walked the ancient paths into the sacred grove. Since these sacred groves are now rare, we are pleased to offer this oracle deck that can bring us closer to the tree angels once more.

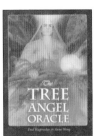

Fred Hageneder, Anne Heng
The Tree Angel Oracle Deck
The Ancient Path into the Sacred Grove
Includes 144-page book and 36 full-color cards
ISBN 978-1-64411-038-6

This oracle set offers a hands-on way to connect with the spiritual wisdom of dragons. Each of the 43 cards features beautiful artwork to allow you to activate dragon energies and use them on an intuitive level. The guidebook details the message of each card and offers meditative journeys into the world of dragons.

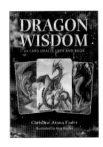

Christine Arana Fader
Dragon Wisdom
43-Card Oracle Deck and Book
Includes 112-page book and 43 full-color cards
ISBN 978-1-64411-108-6

This powerful book with its beautiful illustrations allows you to enter the mystical world of dragons. Once you are ready, it will help you get to know your own dragon, your close personal companion, and to share its invincibility, wisdom, and magic.

Christine Arana Fader
The Little Book of Dragons
Finding your spirit guide
Paperback, full-color throughout, 120 pages
ISBN 978-1-84409-670-1

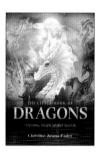

Discover everything you need to know about the luminous infinity symbol. Use the simple exercises contained in this book for decision-making, improving your relationships, reconnecting the analytical and the emotional sides of your brain, and more. The lemniscate can be used in a wide variety of ways.

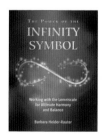

Barbara Heider-Rauter
The Power of the Infinity Symbol
Working with the lemniscate for ultimate harmony and balance
Paperback, full-color throughout, 128 pages
ISBN 978-1-84409-752-4

Both Ho'oponopono, the Hawaiian forgiveness ritual, and family constellation therapy help to heal our relationships with the world around us and bring healing to our inner world. This hands-on book brings together what belongs together, providing beginners with an introduction and easy access to the subject and the more experienced with fresh insights.

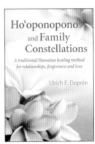

Ulrich Emil Duprée
Ho'oponopono and Family Constellations
A traditional Hawaiian healing method for relationships, forgiveness, and love
Paperback, full-color throughout, 160 pages
ISBN 978-1-84409-717-3

This handy pocket guide presents 40 easy, quick, yet effective ways to boost your energy, rebuild your focus, enhance performance, get better sleep, and bring your life back into balance. Includes simple mental and physical techniques, several recipes, as well as an index of the methods listed according to the desired effect.

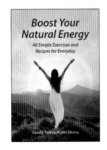

Sandy Taikyu Kuhn Shimu
Boost Your Natural Energy
40 Simple Exercises and Recipes for Everyday
Paperback, full-color throughout, 96 pages
ISBN 978-1-62055-974-1

Disclaimer

The author and publishers accept no liability for the recipes and methods described in this book. Neither the author nor the publishers shall be liable for any damages that may arise from using the tips and advice set out in the book. Consult your doctor, dentist, or alternative practitioner in the event of any health concerns. The methods described do not represent an alternative to therapeutic or medicinal treatment.

For further information and to request a book catalogue contact:
Inner Traditions, One Park Street, Rochester, Vermont 05767

Earthdancer Books is an Inner Traditions imprint.
Phone: +1-800-246-8648, customerservice@innertraditions.com
www.earthdancerbooks.com • www.innertraditions.com

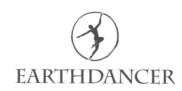

EARTHDANCER

AN INNER TRADITIONS IMPRINT